Advances in Lymphatic Medicine

Edited by Hilal Arnouk

Published in London, United Kingdom

Advances in Lymphatic Medicine
http://dx.doi.org/10.5772/intechopen.1005944
Edited by Hilal Arnouk

Contributors
Abdalqader Aljaradat, Aseel Alashqar, Cédric Zubler, Hilal Arnouk, Jianchun Cui, Joseph Harfouche, Jyothsna Butchireddy, Kenana Altel, Maaweya Jabareen, Marcus Wölffer, Mirela Mariana Roman, Muhammad Al-Sweity, Olivier Leduc, Pierre Bourgeois, Prakash Sivaramakrishnan, Romain Barbieux, Wasef Alhroub, Yang Gao

First published in London, United Kingdom, 2026 by IntechOpen
IntechOpen is the global imprint of INTECHOPEN LIMITED, registered in England and Wales, registration number: 11086078, 167-169 Great Portland Street, London, W1W 5PF, United Kingdom

For EU product safety concerns: IN TECH d.o.o., Prolaz Marije Krucifikse Kozulić 3, 51000 Rijeka, Croatia, info@intechopen.com or visit our website at intechopen.com.

British Library Cataloguing-in-Publication Data
A catalogue record for this book is available from the British Library

Advances in Lymphatic Medicine
Edited by Hilal Arnouk
p. cm.
Print ISBN 978-1-83634-767-5
Online ISBN 978-1-83634-766-8
eBook (PDF) ISBN 978-1-83634-768-2

Meet the editor

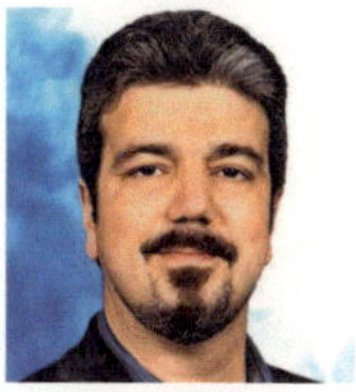

Hilal Arnouk, M. D., Ph.D., is a Professor and the Pathology Discipline Lead at Illinois College of Osteopathic Medicine at The Chicago School. Dr. Arnouk has over three decades of experience in Medical Education and Biomedical Research, with a track record of innovation and leadership of cross-functional teams in the fields of Precision Medicine, Cancer Immunotherapy, Oncology, and Molecular Pathology. Dr. Arnouk received his education and post-doctorate training at Roswell Park Cancer Institute, the State University of New York at Buffalo, the Medical College of Georgia, and the University of Alabama at Birmingham. He has directed research programs as a Principal Investigator in both academic and biotech settings. Additionally, Dr. Arnouk greatly enjoys being an educator and mentor to medical and graduate students.

Contents

Preface

"Our lives are made
In these small hours
These little wonders
These twists and turns of fate
Time falls away
But these small hours
Still remain".

— Little Wonders
Song by Rob Thomas

The lymphatic system is one of the most elusive systems in the human body. It is composed of a network of lymphatic vessels that function as a secondary circulatory system, transporting interstitial fluid and regulating fluid homeostasis. It also contains lymphoid organs, such as the lymph nodes, spleen, appendix, and mucosa-associated lymphoid tissues. The lymphatic system is closely associated with the immune system, as it filters out pathogens and houses phagocytes and lymphocytes that orchestrate innate and adaptive immune responses.

This book is a collaboration between scientists and clinicians that presents the latest developments in lymphatic medicine, including current and emerging imaging and surgical techniques, updates on classification, lymphorrhagia, lymphoma, Castleman Disease, and the concept of sentinel lymph as a gatekeeper of cancer spread. Authors discuss the pathogenesis, diagnosis, and treatment of lymphatic diseases, outlining the advantages and challenges in the field. Additionally, they highlight the role of regenerative medicine in bioengineering new lymphatic structures, including their creation, design, and clinical utility.

I want to thank everyone at IntechOpen publishing for their help with this publication, and I dedicate this book to my family, my colleagues, my mentors, and my students.

Hilal Arnouk, M.D., Ph.D.
Professor and Pathology Discipline Lead,
Illinois College of Osteopathic Medicine at The Chicago School,
Chicago, Illinois, United States

Chapter 1

Introduction to the Sentinel Lymph Node as a Gatekeeper of Cancer Spread Concept

Aseel Alashqar and Hilal Arnouk

Abstract

The first lymph node to receive drainage from a primary tumor is called a sentinel lymph node, acting as a "gatekeeper" for metastatic spread. Surgical techniques have been developed to visualize and biopsy the sentinel lymph node by injecting dyes into the primary tumor to map out the lymphatic flow. The subsequent pathological examination of the resected sentinel lymph nodes can help determine the extent of a cancerous metastatic spread and provide valuable information regarding prognosis and clinical management for patients with various malignancies, including melanoma, breast cancer, gynecologic cancers, and head and neck cancers. Importantly, since these procedures are less invasive than surgical dissections, sentinel lymph node evaluation can reduce the morbidity associated with complete surgical lymph node dissection. The purpose of this chapter is to introduce the concept of the sentinel lymph node and its role in lymphatic medicine, with a focus on its clinical applications across several types of cancer.

Keywords: sentinel lymph node biopsy, sentinel lymph node mapping, metastatic cancer, cancer diagnosis, cancer prognosis, gynecologic cancers, breast cancer, melanoma, lymphatic medicine, lymphatic vessels

1. Introduction

The discovery of the lymphatic system dates back to 1653, when the first lymphatic vessel was described by Bartholin. Over time, further studies revealed the role of the lymphatic system. In the nineteenth century, Rudolf Virchow proposed that lymph nodes act as biological filters. This idea shifted our perception of cancer by establishing the role of lymph nodes in cancer metastasis, thereby suggesting that surgery can be used to manage early stages. This understanding challenged the early Greek prevailing belief that cancer was a local manifestation of a systemic illness. Building on Virchow's theory, William Halsted introduced the radical mastectomy at the end of the nineteenth century, marking a major advance in oncologic surgical treatments [1].

The sentinel lymph node acts as a biological gatekeeper by being the initial site of lymphatic drainage from a primary tumor. It filters tumor cells as they metastasize,

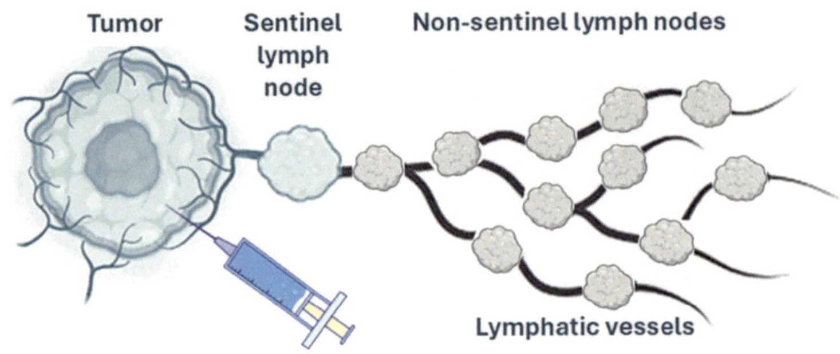

Figure 1.
Schematic depiction of the sentinel node mapping concept, the sentinel lymph node near the tumor is the first site of metastatic spread. Microsoft Office PowerPoint and BioRender software were used to construct this original figure.

and has a unique microenvironment rich in dendritic cells, T cells, and macrophages. This microenvironment plays a key role in immune surveillance and influences tumor progression. Importantly, pathological examination of the sentinel lymph node provides important prognostic information about cancer metastasis to the lymph nodes and recurrence risk, which can help guide treatment plans.

The sentinel lymph node (SLN) is the first lymph node to receive drainage from a primary tumor. SLN mapping and biopsy provide useful information for both treatment planning and prognosis. If a tumor has not yet reached the SLN, in most cases, lymphadenectomy can be omitted, and surgical morbidity is thus avoided [2]. SLN mapping is a critical procedure in the staging of various cancers, including breast cancer, melanoma, gynecologic cancers, and head and neck squamous cell carcinoma. Two prime agents used for this purpose are blue dye, and technetium-99m-labeled tilmanocept (Tc-99m-tilmanocept). The agents are injected into the primary tumor, and the first lymph node to pick up the dye is considered the sentinel lymph node, thus allowing for direct visualization of metastatic spread. Once identified, SLNs are excised and evaluated for pathology, providing information on nodal metastasis, thus decreasing the morbidity associated with complete lymph node dissection (**Figure 1**) [3, 4].

Undoubtedly the history of lymphatic system science has guided our understanding in cancer biology and metastasis, and SLN mapping has become a cornerstone of modern oncologic staging. This chapter explores the clinical application of SLN mapping and biopsies in common malignancies, including breast, melanoma, gynecologic, and head and neck cancers.

2. Breast cancer

Breast cancer remains the most commonly diagnosed cancer in women worldwide [5]. Consequently, prognosis and treatment plans heavily depend on accurate and precise lymph node status assessment [6].

The breast develops from ectodermal tissue during embryogenesis and is essentially an extension of the skin, and thus, its lymphatic drainage follows a similar pattern to the overlying skin. The mammary glands sit between the superficial (subdermal) and deep (subcutaneous) lymphatic networks interconnected by a network of lymphatic vessels [7]. Mammary lymphatics primarily drain to the ipsilateral axilla, however about 3% drain to the internal mammary lymph nodes [8], with even smaller amounts reaching periclavicular, paramammary, intercostal, contralateral breast, or occasionally abdominal lymph nodes [9].

The 2025 American Society of Clinical Oncology (ASCO) guidelines establish sentinel lymph node biopsy (SLNB) as the preferred method for axillary staging in early-stage breast cancer. Axillary lymph node dissection is associated with increased risk of lymphedema, pain, reduced strength, and decreased shoulder range of motion [10]. Thus, SLNB is recognized as a safe and effective procedure that significantly reduces the morbidity associated with axillary lymph node dissection (ALND), particularly in patients who present with clinically node-negative disease [11].

A systematic review and meta-analysis on the impact of SLNB in over 100,000 older female patients with early-stage breast invasive breast cancer demonstrated that positive SLNB findings significantly increase the likelihood of receiving adjuvant chemotherapy and radiation therapy. Specifically, patients with positive SLNB results were 4.6 times more likely to receive chemotherapy and 1.7 times more likely to receive radiation therapy compared to those with negative SLNB results [12]. Thus, SLNB can be used as a valuable tool in guiding treatment plans for patients with breast cancer.

3. Melanoma

Malignant cutaneous melanoma arises from melanocytes and is among the most aggressive forms of skin cancer [13]. Currently, sentinel lymph node biopsy (SLNB) is considered the standard approach for evaluating lymph node involvement in early-stage melanoma. Melanoma staging follows the American Joint Committee on Cancer (AJCC) guidelines, which uses the TNM system to designate the clinical stage [14]. At the time of diagnosis, approximately 84% of cutaneous melanoma cases present as localized disease (stage I–II), 9% show regional lymph node involvement (stage III), and 4% present with distant metastases (stage IV). Importantly, the presence or absence of lymph node metastasis is the key prognostic factor for patients with early-stage melanoma (stage I-II) [15].

SLNB is recommended for patients with a Breslow thickness, or the depth of invasion, of at least 1 mm and should also be considered in tumors 0.8–1.0 mm (with or without ulceration) or even <0.8 mm if risk factors are present. These risk factors include younger age, as patients under 40 have higher SLN positivity rates than older patients, as well as lymphovascular invasion, a positive deep biopsy margin close to 0.8 mm, and high mitotic activity ($\geq$1 mitosis/mm^2) [16]. However, there are certain contraindications to performing SLNB in melanoma patients, including advanced age, poor functional status, evidence of local or systemic spread, prior surgery near the primary tumor or lymph node basin, and comorbidities that may limit life expectancy [17]. It is worth mentioning that with age, the lymphatic system becomes less predictable, making SLNs difficult to detect and ultimately decreasing the accuracy of SLNB [18].

SLNB remains the most critical prognostic tool in cutaneous melanoma, as it helps identify patients at higher risk of recurrence and guide treatment plans. Data collected from a study on SLNB positive melanoma patients showed a decrease in complete lymph node dissection (CLND) alongside an increase in the use of adjuvant systemic therapies between the years 2017 and 2021. While CLND has historically been the standard of care for positive SLNB in cutaneous melanoma, promising data shows that adjuvant therapy is associated with improvements in relapse free survival. Moving forward, it is likely that treatment plans for SLNB positive melanoma will evolve and rely on less invasive adjuvant systemic therapies rather than CLND [19].

Recent studies have expanded the role of SLNB in cutaneous melanoma, particularly regarding its prognostic value and role in risk stratification. Although SLNB has high detection rates, the false negative rate remains at 5–10% mainly in cases with complex lymphatic drainage or thin primary tumors defined by a Breslow thickness of ≤1.0 mm [20]. Because many SLNBs are negative, molecular profiling has emerged as a tool to improve patient selection by analyzing gene expression patterns linked to tumor behavior, including the likelihood of nodal metastasis. Molecular profiling in cutaneous melanoma involves a new method that integrates traditional clinicopathologic features with a 31-gene expression profile (31-GEP) using an artificial intelligence-based neural network algorithm (i31-GEP), which has shown to more accurately stratify the risk of SLN positivity than histologic criteria alone. The algorithm calculates a patient's risk of having a positive SLN, thereby identifying the patients that are more likely to benefit from SLNB [21]. In a recent prospective multicenter study in patients diagnosed with cutaneous melanoma, none of the patients with an i31-GEP–predicted risk below 5% had a positive sentinel lymph node, indicating that SLNB could potentially be avoided in these low-risk individuals [22]. This new approach shows the significance of integrating molecular profiling with traditional clinicopathological parameters to improve the accuracy of SLNB in melanoma.

4. Gynecologic cancers

Endometrial cancer is one of the most common gynecologic malignancies [5] and lymph node involvement serves as an important prognostic factor. The SLN in endometrial cancer is the first lymph node to receive drainage from the uterus, which are typically the external iliac and obturator nodes. The internal iliac, para-aortic, and inguinal nodes can be involved; however, this is less common [23]. Cancer staging can be determined via surgery, which involves a full pelvic and para-aortic lymphadenectomy. This invasive approach is associated with comorbidities including lymphedema, lymphocyst formation [24], and genitofemoral nerve injury [25]. The role of SLN mapping in endometrial cancer was revealed in a recent study that validated SLN mapping by injecting indocyanine green dye into the cervix. Results showed that SLN biopsy achieved a 97.2% sensitivity for detecting nodal metastases compared with complete lymphadenectomy, while significantly reducing surgical morbidity [23]. Thus, SLN mapping is considered a less invasive but accurate alternative for nodal staging.

Similar to endometrial carcinoma, cervical carcinoma relies on sentinel lymph node mapping for staging in early-stage tumors less than 2 cm without apparent nodal involvement [26]. Studies have shown that the majority of SLNs in cervical carcinoma are located in the external iliac, obturator, and internal iliac regions. Interestingly, patient factors such as older age and elevated body mass index (BMI) are associated with a decreased SLN count [27]. Although SLN mapping in cervical cancer follows a technique similar to that used in endometrial cancer, cervical cancer demonstrates a bilateral sentinel node detection rate of 82% in women with early-stage disease, thus indicating that both sides of the pelvis are commonly involved in lymphatic drainage [28].

In contrast, SLN mapping remains a topic of investigation for ovarian carcinoma because of its complex lymphatic drainage [29]. Epithelial ovarian cancer can metastasize through three main pathways; the abdominal pathway, via the infundibulopelvic ligament to para-aortic nodes; the pelvic pathway, via the ovarian ligament toward the iliac vessels and obturator fossa; and the inguinal pathway, via the round ligament of the uterus [30]. Consequently, sentinel lymph nodes can appear in different regions, making SLN mapping more challenging and less reliable compared to endometrial or cervical cancers. Recent studies, however, have shown promising results in using technetium-99m sulfur colloid to detect sentinel lymph nodes in early- stage ovarian cancer, with a detection rate of 100% in one study [31]. These findings suggest that SLN mapping could eventually serve as a less invasive alternative to lymphadenectomy. However, further research regarding oncologic outcomes is required before SLN mapping can become a standard part of ovarian cancer staging.

5. Head and neck cancers

Head and neck squamous-cell carcinoma (HNSCC) is a malignant neoplasm arising from epithelial cells lining the oral cavity, pharynx and larynx. Oral squamous cell carcinoma (OSCC) is the most common type of HNSCC, it most commonly originates in the tongue and frequently metastasizes to cervical lymph nodes [32]. Lymph node involvement in the neck is the most significant prognostic factor in head and neck cancers [33]. Like many other cancers, the presence of nodal metastasis plays a critical role in both staging and guiding treatment plans [34]. In fact, regional lymph node involvement has been shown to reduce the five-year survival rate in head and neck squamous cell carcinoma to approximately 50% [35].

HNSCCs follow the AJCC guidelines for tumor staging, thereby using TNM system where T describes the size of the tumor, N indicates the number, size, and location of affected cervical lymph nodes, and M indicates distant metastasis. Traditionally, elective neck dissection was performed on N0 HNSCC due to a 15–20% risk of lymphatic spread [36], where N0 indicates no lymph node involvement. However, this invasive approach is associated with risk of shoulder dysfunction, lymphedema, sensory deficits, and scarring [37].

One retrospective study on early stage, clinically node negative, oral tongue SCC evaluated SLNB as an alternative to elective neck dissection. Results revealed that SLNB detected lymph node metastases in 24.6% of patients, thus supporting the role of SLNB as a reliable method for detecting early metastasis [38].

6. Discussion, conclusions, and future directions

Recent scientific advancements continue to reshape the future of sentinel lymph node biopsy, with the goal of improving diagnostic accuracy while minimizing procedural morbidity. New hybrid tracers such as indocyanine green–^{99m}Tc nanocolloid have demonstrated higher detection rates than conventional radiocolloid, mainly in endometrial cancer with complex lymphatic drainage to the para-aortic lymph nodes [39].

Superparamagnetic iron oxide (SPIO) nanoparticles have also emerged as a radiation-free alternative for SLN mapping, playing an important role in identifying sentinel lymph nodes in patients with clinically node-negative breast cancer. A recent meta-analysis for a large cohort of patients demonstrated that SPIO-guided SLNB is at least as effective, and in some cases more effective, than standard radiocolloid-based techniques, with the added benefit of being non-radioactive [40]. Furthermore, SPIO may potentially play a role as an alternative tracer for SLN mapping in patients with cutaneous melanoma. A recent systematic review and meta-analysis found that SPIO-guided SLN biopsy had a sensitivity of nearly 94%, thus providing detection rates comparable to the conventional radioisotope and dye method [41].

Moreover, artificial intelligence (AI) has shown a promising role in digital pathology for evaluating SLNs. In melanoma, a recent study showed that a deep learning model could accurately distinguish between positive and negative SLNs, correctly identifying a positive node 96.5% of the time. This performance is comparable to that of expert dermatopathologists [42]. In breast cancer, another large study analyzed over 32,000 sentinel lymph node slides and found that when pathologists used AI as a support tool, their ability to detect metastases improved from about 74.5 to 93.5%, while the time needed to review each slide dropped by more than half [43]. As the field of digital pathology continues to grow, AI-based analysis may be a useful prognostic tool for cancers where the nodal involvement is difficult to assess, such as in early-stage melanoma. AI can potentially help pathologists in detecting micrometastasis and improve efficiency in detecting SLNs in different types of cancers.

It is important to note that the role of the sentinel lymph node evaluation varies across different cancer types due to differences in tumor biology and pathogenesis. In early-stage breast cancer, sentinel lymph node biopsy (SLNB) acts as a minimally invasive staging tool that has practically replaced axillary lymph node dissection (ALND). SLNB can accurately identify nodal metastasis, and large clinical trials have shown that omitting axillary lymph node dissection in patients with limited SLN involvement reduces morbidity without affecting long-term survival [44]. In melanoma, SLNB is primarily an important predictor of prognosis as the SLN status is closely associated with disease-specific survival, with a negative SLN predicting significantly longer melanoma-specific survival. Thus, SLNB plays an important role in risk stratification and in guiding follow-up and adjuvant therapy decisions [45]. Importantly, While SLNB can detect occult metastases in both types of cancer, the clinical management implications differ. In breast cancer, SLNB findings influence decisions about surgery and adjuvant therapy, whereas in melanoma, SLN positivity informs prognosis and staging rather than providing a clear overall survival benefit. This comparison highlights that the clinical utility of the SLNB depends on the tumor type, biology and pathogenesis. Thus, underscoring the importance of interpreting SLNB results within the context of the underlying malignancy.

In conclusion, the concept of the sentinel lymph node has changed our approach to cancer staging and surgical intervention, especially for breast, melanoma, gynecologic, and head and neck cancers. Overall, SLN mapping and biopsy provide important prognostic information and can improve patient outcomes by detecting early nodal metastasis. These procedures are less invasive than surgical dissections and lymphadenectomies, and they are not associated with complications such as lymphedema, thus improving patient's quality of life. Unfortunately, these techniques play a limited role in malignancies with complex lymphatic drainage, such as ovarian cancer. Ongoing research aims to improve the accuracy and use of SLNB by developing novel tracers, employing molecular profiling, and incorporating AI and digital pathology. These advances can potentially improve the detection of micrometastases and further expand the role of SLNB across a wider range of cancers. Overall, sentinel lymph node mapping and biopsy will continue to play an important role in cancer management.

Author details

Aseel Alashqar[1] and Hilal Arnouk[2]*

1 Chicago College of Osteopathic Medicine, Midwestern University, Illinois, United States

2 Illinois College of Osteopathic Medicine at The Chicago School, Illinois, United States

*Address all correspondence to: harnou@midwestern.edu

References

[1] Halsted WS. I. The results of operations for the cure of cancer of the breast performed at the Johns Hopkins Hospital from June, 1889, to January, 1894. Annals of Surgery. 1894;**20**(5):497-555. DOI: 10.1097/00000658-189407000-00075

[2] Dogan NU, Dogan S, Favero G, Köhler C, Dursun P. The basics of sentinel lymph node biopsy: Anatomical and pathophysiological considerations and clinical aspects. Journal of Oncology. 2019;**2019**:3415630. DOI: 10.1155/2019/3415630

[3] Tausch C, Baege A, Rageth C. Mapping lymph nodes in cancer management - Role of (99m)Tc-tilmanocept injection. Oncotargets and Therapy. 2014;**7**:1151-1158. DOI: 10.2147/OTT.S50394

[4] Kern KA. Sentinel lymph node mapping in breast cancer using subareolar injection of blue dye. Journal of the American College of Surgeons. 1999;**189**(6):539-545. DOI: 10.1016/s1072-7515(99)00200-8

[5] Siegel RL, Kratzer TB, Giaquinto AN, Sung H, Jemal A. Cancer statistics, 2025. CA: A Cancer Journal for Clinicians. 2025;**75**(1):10-45. DOI: 10.3322/caac.21871

[6] Zurrida S, Veronesi U. Milestones in breast cancer treatment. The Breast Journal. 2015;**21**(1):3-12. DOI: 10.1111/tbj.12361

[7] Suami H, Pan WR, Mann GB, Taylor GI. The lymphatic anatomy of the breast and its implications for sentinel lymph node biopsy: A human cadaver study. Annals of Surgical Oncology. 2008;**15**(3):863-871. DOI: 10.1245/s10434-007-9709-9

[8] Turner-Warwick RT. The lymphatics of the breast. British Journal of Surgery. 1959;**46**(200):574-582. DOI: 10.1002/bjs.18004620004

[9] Estourgie SH, Nieweg OE, Olmos RA, Rutgers EJ, Kroon BB. Lymphatic drainage patterns from the breast. Annals of Surgery. 2004;**239**(2):232-237. DOI: 10.1097/01.sla.0000109156.26378.90

[10] Che Bakri NA, Kwasnicki RM, Khan N, Ghandour O, Lee A, Grant Y, et al. Impact of axillary lymph node dissection and sentinel lymph node biopsy on upper limb morbidity in breast cancer patients: A systematic review and meta-analysis. Annals of Surgery. 2023;**277**(4):572-580. DOI: 10.1097/SLA.0000000000005671

[11] Park KU, Somerfield MR, Anne N, Brackstone M, Conlin AK, Couto HL, et al. Sentinel lymph node biopsy in early-stage breast cancer: ASCO guideline update. Journal of Clinical Oncology: Official Journal of the American Society of Clinical Oncology. 2025;**43**(14):1720-1741. DOI: 10.1200/JCO-25-00099

[12] Daly GR, Dowling GP, Said M, Qasem Y, Hembrecht S, Calpin GG, et al. Impact of sentinel lymph node biopsy on management of older women with clinically node-negative, early-stage, ER+/HER2-, invasive breast cancer: A systematic review and meta-analysis. Clinical Breast Cancer. 2024;**24**(8):e681-e688.e1. DOI: 10.1016/j.clbc.2024.07.012

[13] Leonardi GC, Falzone L, Salemi R, Zanghì A, Spandidos DA, Mccubrey JA, et al. Cutaneous melanoma: From pathogenesis to therapy (review). International Journal of Oncology.

2018;**52**(4):1071-1080. DOI: 10.3892/ijo.2018.4287

[14] Keung EZ, Gershenwald JE. The eighth edition American Joint Committee on Cancer (AJCC) melanoma staging system: Implications for melanoma treatment and care. Expert Review of Anticancer Therapy. 2018;**18**(8):775-784. DOI: 10.1080/14737140.2018.1489246

[15] Tardelli E, Mazzarri S, Rubello D, Gennaro M, Fantechi L, Duce V, et al. Sentinel lymph node biopsy in cutaneous melanoma. Clinical Nuclear Medicine. 2016;**41**(12):e498-e507. DOI: 10.1097/RLU.0000000000001370

[16] Branisteanu DE, Cozmin M, Porumb-Andrese E, Branisteanu D, Toader MP, Iosep D, et al. Sentinel lymph node biopsy in cutaneous melanoma, a clinical point of view. Medicina (Kaunas, Lithuania). 2022;**58**(11):1589. DOI: 10.3390/medicina58111589

[17] Swetter SM, Thompson JA, Albertini MR, Barker CA, Baumgartner J, Boland G, et al. NCCN guidelines® insights: Melanoma: Cutaneous, version 2.2021. Journal of the National Comprehensive Cancer Network: JNCCN. 2021;**19**(4):364-376. DOI: 10.6004/jnccn.2021.0018

[18] Sinnamon AJ, Neuwirth MG, Bartlett EK, Zaheer S, Etherington MS, Xu X, et al. Predictors of false negative sentinel lymph node biopsy in trunk and extremity melanoma. Journal of Surgical Oncology. 2017;**116**(7):848-855. DOI: 10.1002/jso.24743

[19] Zietek M, Teterycz P, Wierzbicki J, Jankowski M, Las-Jankowska M, Zegarski W, et al. The current treatment trends and survival patterns in melanoma patients with positive sentinel lymph node biopsy (SLNB): A multicenter nationwide study. Cancers. 2023;**15**(10):2667. DOI: 10.3390/cancers15102667

[20] Allard-Coutu A, Dobson V, Schmitz E, Shah H, Nessim C. The evolution of the sentinel node biopsy in melanoma. Life. 2023;**13**(2):489. DOI: 10.3390/life13020489

[21] Whitman ED, Koshenkov VP, Gastman BR, Lewis D, Hsueh EC, Pak H, et al. Integrating 31-gene expression profiling with clinicopathologic features to optimize cutaneous melanoma sentinel lymph node metastasis prediction. JCO Precision Oncology. 2021;**5**:PO.21.00162. DOI: 10.1200/PO.21.00162

[22] Guenther JM, Ward A, Martin BJ, Cripe M, Sharma R, Leong SP, et al. A prospective, multicenter analysis of the integrated 31-gene expression profile test for sentinel lymph node biopsy (i31-GEP for SLNB) test demonstrates reduced number of unnecessary SLNBs in patients with cutaneous melanoma. World Journal of Surgical Oncology. 2025;**23**(1):5. DOI: 10.1186/s12957-024-03640-x

[23] Rossi EC, Kowalski LD, Scalici J, Cantrell L, Schuler K, Hanna RK, et al. A comparison of sentinel lymph node biopsy to lymphadenectomy for endometrial cancer staging (FIRES trial): A multicentre, prospective, cohort study. The Lancet. Oncology. 2017;**18**(3):384-392. DOI: 10.1016/S1470-2045(17)30068-2

[24] Abu-Rustum NR, Alektiar K, Iasonos A, Lev G, Sonoda Y, Aghajanian C, et al. The incidence of symptomatic lower-extremity lymphedema following treatment of uterine corpus malignancies: A 12-year experience at Memorial Sloan-Kettering Cancer Center. Gynecologic Oncology. 2006;**103**(2):714-718. DOI: 10.1016/j.ygyno.2006.03.055

[25] Cardosi RJ, Cox CS, Hoffman MS. Postoperative neuropathies after major pelvic surgery. Obstetrics and Gynecology. 2002;**100**(2):240-244. DOI: 10.1016/s0029-7844(02)02052-5

[26] Diaz-Feijoo B, Temprana-Salvador J, Franco-Camps S, Manrique S, Colás E, Pérez-Benavente A, et al. Clinical management of early-stage cervical cancer: The role of sentinel lymph node biopsy in tumors ≤2 cm. European Journal of Obstetrics, Gynecology, and Reproductive Biology. 2019;**241**:30-34. DOI: 10.1016/j.ejogrb.2019.07.038

[27] Wuntakal R, Papadopoulos AJ, Montalto SA, Perovic M, Coutts M, Devaja O. Location of sentinel lymph node in cervical carcinoma and factors associated with unilateral detection. International Journal of Gynecological Cancer: Official Journal of the International Gynecological Cancer Society. 2015;**25**(9):1663-1668. DOI: 10.1097/IGC.0000000000000539

[28] Sponholtz SE, Mogensen O, Hildebrandt MG, Schledermann D, Parner E, Markauskas A, et al. Sentinel lymph node mapping in early-stage cervical cancer - A national prospective multicenter study (SENTIREC trial). Gynecologic Oncology. 2021;**162**(3):546-554. DOI: 10.1016/j.ygyno.2021.06.018

[29] Wang T, Xu Y, Shao W, Wang C. Sentinel lymph node mapping: Current applications and future perspectives in gynecology malignant tumors. Frontiers in Medicine. 2022;**9**:922585. DOI: 10.3389/fmed.2022.922585

[30] Kleppe M, Kraima AC, Kruitwagen RF, Van Gorp T, Smit NN, van Munsteren JC, et al. Understanding lymphatic drainage pathways of the ovaries to predict sites for sentinel nodes in ovarian cancer. International Journal of Gynecological Cancer: Official Journal of the International Gynecological Cancer Society. 2015;**25**(8):1405-1414. DOI: 10.1097/IGC.0000000000000514

[31] Heda A, Rajaram S, Bahadur A, Gaurav A, Dhingra VK, Chowdhury N, et al. Sentinel lymph node detection in early-stage ovarian cancer using radionuclide technetium-99m Sulfur colloid - A feasibility study. Indian Journal of Nuclear Medicine: IJNM: The Official Journal of the Society of Nuclear Medicine, India. 2025;**40**(1):16-21. DOI: 10.4103/ijnm.ijnm_149_24

[32] Woolgar JA, Rogers SN, Lowe D, Brown JS, Vaughan ED. Cervical lymph node metastasis in oral cancer: The importance of even microscopic extracapsular spread. Oral Oncology. 2003;**39**(2):130-137. DOI: 10.1016/s1368-8375(02)00030-1

[33] Yamauchi K, Kogashiwa Y, Nakamura T, Moro Y, Nagafuji H, Kohno N. Diagnostic evaluation of sentinel lymph node biopsy in early head and neck squamous cell carcinoma: A meta-analysis. Head & Neck. 2015;**37**(1):127-133. DOI: 10.1002/hed.23526

[34] Demir D. The role of sentinel lymph node biopsy in head and neck cancers and its application areas. Turkish Archives of Otorhinolaryngology. 2016;**54**(1):35-38. DOI: 10.5152/tao.2016.1129

[35] Layland MK, Sessions DG, Lenox J. The influence of lymph node metastasis in the treatment of squamous cell carcinoma of the oral cavity, oropharynx, larynx, and hypopharynx: N0 versus N+. The Laryngoscope. 2005;**115**:629-639. DOI: 10.1097/01.mlg.0000161338.54515.b1

[36] Finegersh A, Moss WJ, Saddawi-Konefka R, Faraji F, Coffey CS,

Califano JA, et al. Meta-analysis of risk of occult lymph node metastasis in the irradiated, clinically N0 neck. Head & Neck. 2020;**42**(9):2355-2363. DOI: 10.1002/hed.26248

[37] Schiefke F, Akdemir M, Weber A, Akdemir D, Singer S, Frerich B. Function, postoperative morbidity, and quality of life after cervical sentinel node biopsy and after selective neck dissection. Head & Neck. 2009;**31**(4):503-512. DOI: 10.1002/hed.21001

[38] Ionna F, Pavone E, Aversa C, Maffia F, Spinelli R, Carraturo E, et al. Sentinel lymph node biopsy (SLNB) for early-stage head and neck squamous-cell carcinoma of the tongue: Twenty years of experience at I.N.T. "G.Pascale". Cancers. 2024;**16**(6):1153. DOI: 10.3390/cancers16061153

[39] Sánchez-Izquierdo N, Vidal-Sicart S, Campos F, Torné A, Angeles MA, Migliorelli F, et al. Detection of the sentinel lymph node with hybrid tracer (ICG-[^{99m}Tc]Tc-albumin nanocolloid) in intermediate- and high-risk endometrial cancer: A feasibility study. EJNMMI Research. 2021;**11**(1):123. DOI: 10.1186/s13550-021-00863-x

[40] Liu P, Tan J, Song Y, Huang K, Zhang Q, Xie H. The application of magnetic nanoparticles for sentinel lymph node detection in clinically node-negative breast cancer patients: A systemic review and meta-analysis. Cancers. 2022;**14**(20):5034. DOI: 10.3390/cancers14205034

[41] Taqi K, Jonsson EL, Assadzad GE, Stockley C, Bains I, Temple-Oberle C. Superparamagnetic iron oxide tracer: A magnetic match to gold standard in melanoma sentinel lymph node biopsy- A systematic review and meta-analysis. Journal of Surgical Oncology. 2025;**132**(5):860-868. DOI: 10.1002/jso.70086

[42] Siarov J, Siarov A, Kumar D, Paoli J, Mölne J, Neittaanmäki N. Deep learning model shows pathologist-level detection of sentinel node metastasis of melanoma and intra-nodal nevi on whole slide images. Frontiers in Medicine. 2024;**11**:1418013. DOI: 10.3389/fmed.2024.1418013

[43] Retamero JA, Gulturk E, Bozkurt A, Liu S, Gorgan M, Moral L, et al. Artificial intelligence helps pathologists increase diagnostic accuracy and efficiency in the detection of breast cancer lymph node metastases. The American Journal of Surgical Pathology. 2024;**48**(7):846-854. DOI: 10.1097/PAS.0000000000002248

[44] Krag DN, Anderson SJ, Julian TB, Brown AM, Harlow SP, Costantino JP, et al. Sentinel-lymph-node resection compared with conventional axillary-lymph-node dissection in clinically node-negative patients with breast cancer: Overall survival findings from the NSABP B-32 randomised phase 3 trial. The Lancet. Oncology. 2010;**11**(10):927-933. DOI: 10.1016/S1470-2045(10)70207-2

[45] Wong SL, Faries MB, Kennedy EB, Agarwala SS, Akhurst TJ, Ariyan C, et al. Sentinel lymph node biopsy and Management of Regional Lymph Nodes in melanoma: American Society of Clinical Oncology and Society of Surgical Oncology clinical practice guideline update. Journal of Clinical Oncology: Official Journal of the American Society of Clinical Oncology. 2018;**36**(4):399-413. DOI: 10.1200/JCO.2017.75.7724

Chapter 2

Advances in Lymphatic Imaging for Sentinel Lymph Node Identification in Oncologic Surgery

Marcus Wölffer and Cédric Zubler

Abstract

As an integral part of the TNM staging system, lymph node status represents a crucial prognostic factor in many malignancies. Consequently, sentinel lymph node (SLN) biopsy is part of the standard of care for several tumor entities. Technetium (Tc)-based lymphoscintigraphy currently serves as the gold standard to identify SLNs. However, disadvantages have led to the emergence of alternative modalities for lymphatic imaging and SLN identification. This chapter provides a full overview of the latest technical developments and imaging options available for this procedure across malignancies and analyzes the advantages as well as limitations of each method. One of the most used and successful alternative techniques is indocyanine green (ICG). Approaches such as SPECT-CT or hybrid approaches, combining ICG and Tc, serve as adjuncts or optimize individual techniques. More recently investigated techniques include carbon nanoparticles, superparamagnetic iron oxide nanoparticles, contrast-enhanced ultrasound, and multispectral optoacoustic tomographic imaging.

Keywords: sentinel lymph node biopsy, dermato-oncology, gynecologic oncology, urologic oncology, melanoma, technetium-based lymphoscintigraphy, indocyanine green, hybrid tracers, carbon nanoparticles, superparamagnetic iron oxide, contrast-enhanced ultrasound, SPECT-CT, multispectral optoacoustic tomographic imaging

1. Introduction

Various malignancies metastasize through the lymphatic system. For these tumors, the concept of sentinel lymph nodes (SLN) was proposed. A SLN is the first lymph node draining the local site of the primary tumor and therefore acts as the first filter potentially reached by metastatic cells. In the case of lymphatic metastases, the SLN would be the earliest possible site where malignant cells could be detected. Determining the status of the SLN allows for staging according to the TNM classification. Since the introduction of cutaneous melanoma by Morton et al. [1], identifying and examining the SLN has now become a standard of care procedure in various malignancies. These include but are not limited to breast cancer, melanoma, head and neck malignancies, gastric cancer, colon cancer, uterine cancer as well as vulvar cancer [2].

The status of SLNs has been proven to be one of the most important factors for oncologic prognosis in frequently occurring malignancies such as breast cancer or melanoma [3]. It allows for adequate histological staging according to the current guidelines of the 8th edition UICC/AJCC TNM melanoma staging system [4]. Usually, it also has direct consequences for further oncologic treatment; for example, a positive SLN in otherwise clinically non-metastatic cutaneous melanoma patients warrants the initiation of adjuvant therapy with immune checkpoint inhibitors or targeted therapy [3].

Substantial debate persists on the therapeutic value of the SLN biopsy (SLNB) surgery in addition to its above-mentioned diagnostic and prognostic value. Some authors have argued that SLNB provides long-term regional control of the lymph node basin after positive SLN [5]. Contrary to that, other studies have demonstrated that even immediate complete lymph node dissection after a positive SLNB does not increase melanoma-specific survival [6]. Furthermore, no significant difference in overall survival was found between false-negative and true-positive patients [7].

Regardless of this debate, the diagnostic and prognostic value is assured, and SLNB might become even more relevant in the light of increasing success of neoadjuvant immunotherapy options [8] and the tendency to use adjuvant immunotherapy in earlier tumor stages, such as stage III melanoma [9].

Historically, various methods have been tried to ascertain the relevant SLN tissue. With a sensitivity of only 78% in the case of axillary lymph nodes [10], ultrasound-guided fine needle aspiration biopsy does not exclude metastatic disease with a satisfying accuracy and is therefore not considered a safe option. Removing the lymph node as a whole solves two issues: it allows for the detection of micrometastases that often only occupy small parts of the affected lymph node and avoids tumor seeding potentially associated with partial biopsy of the affected tissue. Therefore, surgical excisional biopsy has become the standard of care in SLNB.

The desired precision of the SLNB poses a significant challenge to surgeons. In most malignancies, typical SLN basin locations can be assumed preoperatively. In endometrial or cervical cancer, for instance, those would be external iliac, obturator, or pelvic lymph node basins [11]. However, up to 5% of SLNs might be located in an unusual location outside established lymph node basins [12]. Furthermore, SLNB in head and neck malignancies in particular is notoriously difficult, with unpredictable drainage patterns leading to multiple or bilateral basins [13]. Additionally, even after the relevant lymph node basin is identified, the challenge remains to find the relevant SLN among often more than 10 non-SLNs during the surgical procedure [14].

Because of this, surgeons depend on preoperative radiological and/or intraoperative visual guidance in order to both identify the SLN basin and the correct SLN within that basin.

Regardless of the method chosen to identify the SLN, the surgical procedure is similar. Depending on the tumor entity, surgery is performed either together with primary excision (e.g., breast cancer) or second resection (e.g., melanoma). The SLN basin is identified and the patient positioned accordingly. Depending on the location of the primary tumor, several potential SLNs can be identified in different basins. The surgical site is disinfected and draped. After the incision, the basin is searched for the SLN under visual or technology-based guidance. The SLN is excised using no-touch technique, and all connected lymphatic vessels are clipped or coagulated. The operation is finished by hemostasis and layered wound closure. Patients can mobilize immediately according to their symptoms.

Technetium-based lymphoscintigraphy (Tc-based LS) is a well-established standard of care for the identification of SLNs [15]. However, it is associated with several disadvantages, which have led to the emergence of a plethora of alternative detection modalities. The optimal lymphatic imaging method should be inexpensive, readily available in all parts of the world, free of adverse events, easy to learn, and identify all SLNs in every patient preoperatively, that is, before skin incision.

This chapter is intended to provide an overview of the latest technical advances and clinically available imaging options for identifying SLNs across different malignancies, including an analysis of advantages and limitations of these methods.

2. Lymphatic imaging techniques for sentinel lymph node biopsy

2.1 Technetium-based lymphoscintigraphy

Technetium-based lymphoscintigraphy (Tc-based LS) represents the gold standard technique in SLNB to date and is widely used for different malignancies. With this approach, radiotracers are used to produce gamma emissions which are registered by a gamma-counting probe or a gamma camera. Different radiotracers are available today, including Tc-99m-pertechnetate-labeled colloids or Tc-99m-tilmanocept [16]. Larger radiotracers drain to and accumulate in lymph nodes and therefore present optimal characteristics for SLN identification. The generally accepted cut-off for optimal size is >40 nm [17]. There is no international consensus on the optimal protocol for Tc-based LS in SLNB. Injections are typically done some hours before surgery by the Department of Nuclear Medicine. Injection doses range from 3.7 MBq in melanoma to 370 MBq in breast cancer. For melanoma, several intradermal injections of 0.1 ml each are performed peritumorally, whereas for breast cancer, subdermal, periareolar or peritumoral injections are performed [16]. Immediately after injection, dynamic imaging is performed over 20–30 minutes to visualize the drainage pattern to the SLN. Hereafter, static imaging is performed with a gamma camera to localize the identified nodes in three dimensions [18]. Depending on the location of the primary tumor, imaging is performed on all possible drainage locations (see **Figure 1**). After visualization of SLNs, a gamma-counting probe is used to locate SLNs and mark the overlaying skin [16]. The surgeon is provided with the LS results before the operation to ensure adequate positioning of the patient during the procedure. Intraoperatively, the marked location of the SLN is confirmed by placing the gamma probe on the patient's skin to identify the area with the highest activity. The incision is carried out and the gamma probe is intermittently used to guide dissection and identify the SLN within the fat of the lymph node basin. After excision of the SLN, the gamma probe is used to detect residual counts in the operative field and potentially remove additional SLNs. While different definitions exist, it is usually recommended that any lymph node presenting a count rate of at least 10% of the hottest SLN should be removed [18]. Since Tc is a colorless tracer, it is often combined with preoperative injection of blue dye to provide the surgeon with some additional visual guidance after incision and thereby increase identification rates. Several different blue dyes are used, and injection techniques again vary depending on the tumor entity. Methylene Blue has been found to be superior to Iso-sulfan Blue or Patent Blue concerning false-negative rate (FNR) [19].

Since its introduction several decades ago, medical professionals have accumulated experience with Tc-based LS. The possibility of combining preoperative imaging

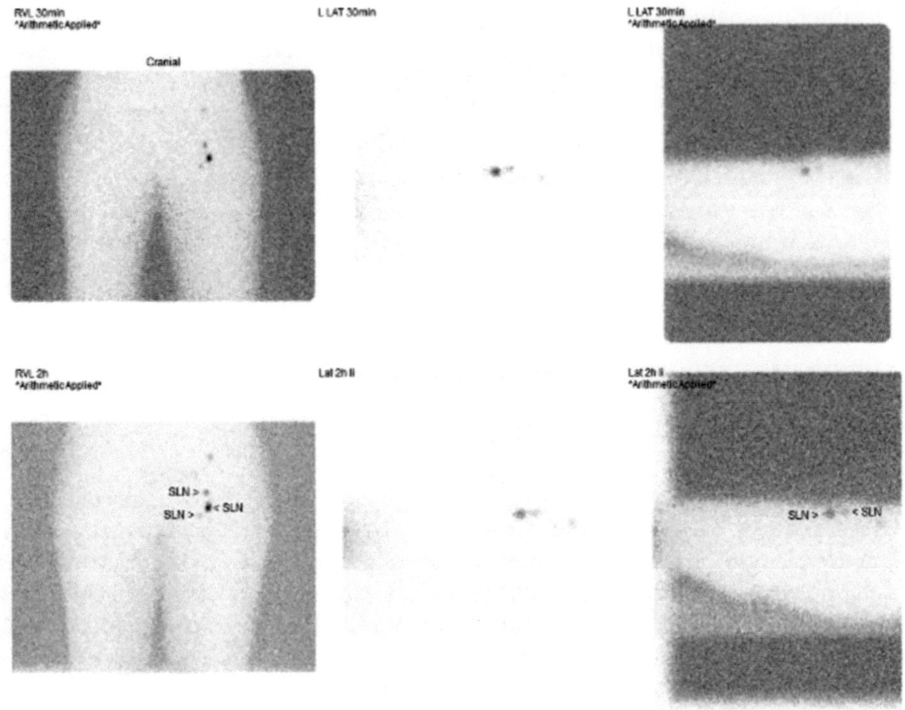

Figure 1.
Technetium-based lymphoscintigraphy with depiction of three SLNs in the left femoral and inguinal basin for a patient with malignant melanoma of the left medial thigh. Furthermore, downstream lymph nodes in the left iliac external basin are visible.

with intraoperative guidance allows precise surgical planning. An incomparable number of studies among SLNB techniques have consistently demonstrated its high detection rates of over 95%. In a meta-analysis of cutaneous melanoma patients, 97% of metastatic patients, 97% of SLNs, and 97% of metastatic SLNs were identified by Tc [20]. Further improvements take place today with the introduction of novel radiotracers, which cause less injection pain and radiation exposure, as well as offer an optimized SLN retention [17]. In a meta-analysis of breast cancer patients, the standard of care Tc-99m-labeled nanocolloid human serum albumin was compared to Tc-99m-tilmanocept. While the first reached a localization rate of 95.91%, the latter demonstrated a rate of 99.99% [21].

Nevertheless, the LS technique also has several disadvantages. Cost analyses have shown the poor cost-effectiveness of this modality when taking into account travel expenses, contrast medium costs and training of hospital staff [22]. Even if it may be low, a radioactive burden exists for medical professionals and patients alike [23]. Tc-based LS is also lacking availability in developing countries, where SLNB is therefore often impossible or difficult to perform [24]. Furthermore, the practical detection of SLNs using Tc-based LS has its own limitations. The shine-through effect, a visual disturbance near the primary tumor caused by radioactive background signals around the site of injection [25], has been reported to reach 11 cm from the primary tumor in the case of breast cancer [26]. This might explain the high FNR of Tc-based LS found in head and neck melanoma patients [27]. Additionally, studies have shown that Tc-based SLNB results in high sampling rates of SLNs without resulting in a correspondingly high number of identified metastatic SLNs or patients compared to indocyanine green (ICG), which might lead to increased incidence of postoperative complications [20]. In some malignancies, Tc has been found to be inferior to other diagnostic approaches. A meta-analysis reviewing its use in patients with cervical cancer showed that while Tc had an overall detection rate of 95%, it only demonstrated a bilateral detection rate of 63%, proving to be inferior to ICG for both outcomes [28].

2.2 SPECT-CT

Single-photon emission computed tomography with integrated computed tomography (SPECT-CT) includes a low-dose CT system and a gamma camera. Images captured by these two modalities are merged in a hybrid, three-dimensional image [29], with the possibility of quantitatively analyzing radioactivity count thresholds to avoid resection of non-metastatic lymph nodes [30]. Today, it is a well-established technique with wide application in nuclear medicine departments and often used as an adjunct in the case of unclear results during Tc-based LS. Especially in the head and neck area, SPECT-CT might provide the surgeon with additional, crucial information about SLNs such as anatomical relation to important structures or precise location in lymph node levels (see **Figures 2** and **3**). SPECT-CT has been shown to allow for more accurate placement of incisions and a more efficient dissection with less morbidity [31]. In complex anatomical regions such as the head and neck, SPECT-CT has been reported to significantly increase the likelihood of identifying a positive SLN, especially for SLNs located in the proximity of the primary tumor or additional basins [32]. In patients with trunk melanoma, SPECT-CT located significantly more SLNs than LS, revealed additional drainage regions necessitating a modification of the surgical approach, and corrected false-positive and false-negative results of LS. Sensitivity of SPECT-CT was 98.6% compared to 95.1% for LS [33]. SPECT-CT may also reduce the FNR. Indeed, it has been shown to identify a significantly higher number of SLNs and metastatic SLNs per patient as

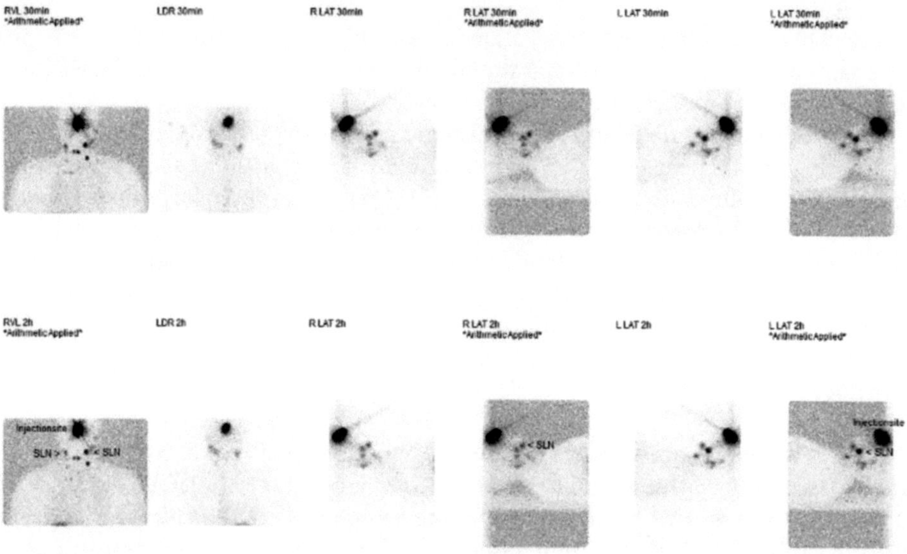

Figure 2.
Technetium-based lymphoscintigraphy with depiction of several bilateral cervical SLNs for a patient with malignant melanoma of the right nasal bridge.

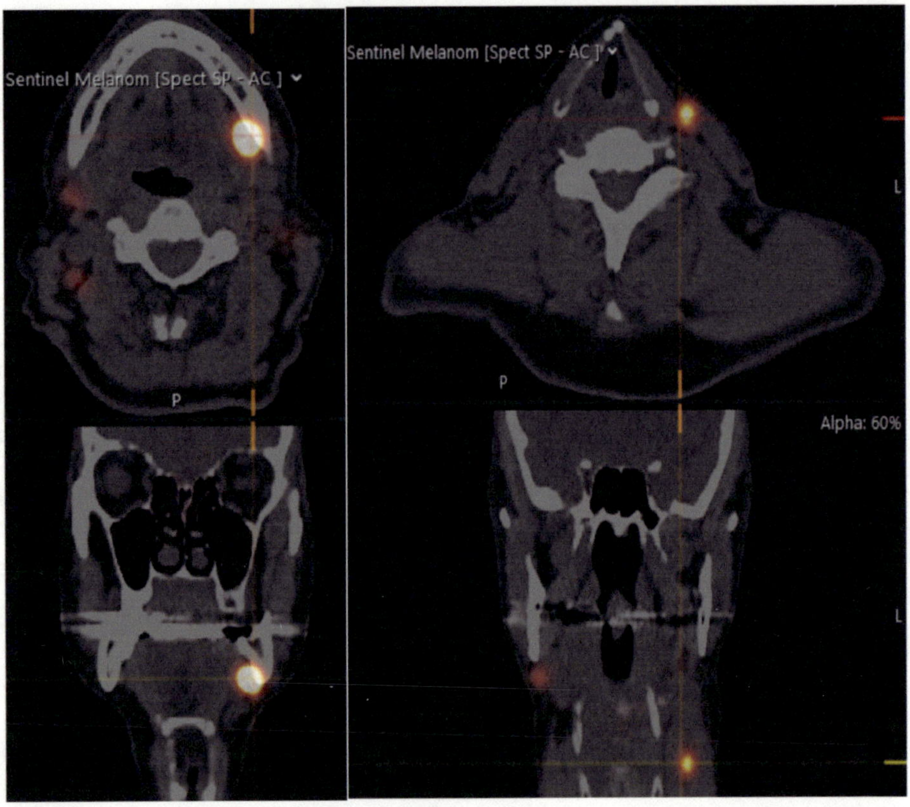

Figure 3.
For the same patient as in **Figure 2**, *transaxial and coronal SPECT-CT images. The comparison to* **Figure 2** *highlights the additional information regarding the exact anatomical location and relation to other structures, which influences surgical planning.*

compared to the standard technique, allowing for a higher rate of disease-free survival. In the same study, a FNR of 6.8% was found for the SPECT-CT group and 23.8% for the standard technique group [31].

Recent technological advancements also include the introduction of freehand SPECT which could be used in the operation room. This technique allows an intraoperative three-dimensional visualization [34]. Previous authors have compared freehand SPECT with conventional gamma probe in breast cancer SLNB. Freehand SPECT was associated with the identification of more nodes per patient and a shorter operating time, even in obese patients [35]. While it increases spatial resolution, its disadvantages include a high radiation exposure [17].

2.3 Indocyanine green

Since Tc-based LS presents the disadvantages mentioned above, authors have strived to find alternative and optimized contrast agents for SLNB. One of the most studied and successful of these is indocyanine green (ICG), a fluorescent molecule tricarbocyanine dye. It absorbs light emitted with a wavelength of 760 nm and reemits it at a higher wavelength on the near-infrared spectrum. This emission can be identified by a near-infrared fluorescence (NIRFI) camera in the operation room which allows for localization of SLNs (see **Figure 4**) [17]. Generally, 0.25 ml of ICG

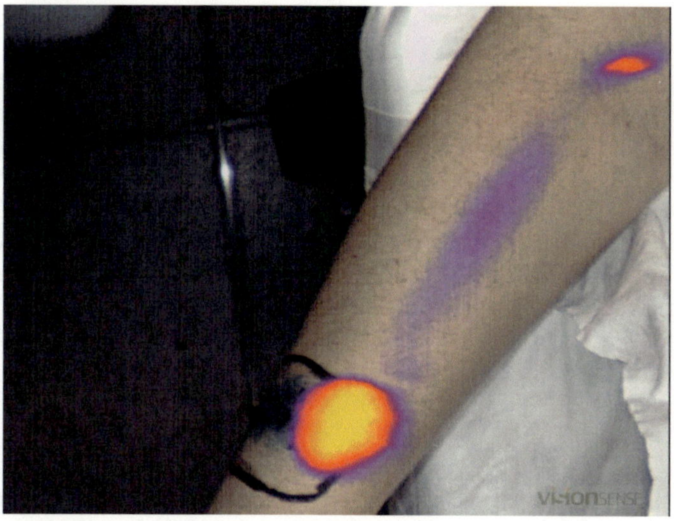

Figure 4.
Indocyanine green-based near-infrared fluorescence imaging with fluorescence captured at the site of injection at the distal forearm, along the lymphatic drainage and at the cubital SLN.

are injected intradermally in four quadrants around the primary tumor. Upon administration, ICG binds with albumin in the extracellular fluid, which is then drained by the lymphatic channels. Drainage and accumulation in the SLN can then be observed in real time during roughly the next 15 minutes. One of the most commonly used camera systems is the SPY Elite (LifeCell Corp, Branchburg, NJ) [36].

No frequent adverse events have been reported yet [37] and ICG presents a very low risk for anaphylactoid reactions (0.05%) in contrast to blue dye. In addition to the transcutaneous visualization using the NIRFI camera, ICG is also visible after incision, thus facilitating dissection for the surgeon. It enables an easier dissection when compared to blue dye as it stains less surrounding tissue and causes no tattooing [36]. The real-time visualization of SLNs may improve operating room efficiency, and the lack of need for a nuclear medicine department results in lower costs and avoided radiation exposure [38, 39].

However, several disadvantages complicate the widespread introduction of ICG in medical practice. The acquisition of the NIRFI machine and training of medical professionals is a significant investment and the learning curve is considerable [20]. The main disadvantage remains the method's superficial tissue penetration, with a transcutaneous visibility of 1 cm [40] to 2 cm [41] only. This explains reported limiting factors for SLNB with ICG such as high BMI [42] and axillary lymph node fields [43]. Previous authors have also pointed out the lack of standardization of the technique with varying location of injection, amount of ICG injected or camera system used [39].

In terms of oncologic safety, studies have compared the accuracy of ICG and Tc in breast cancer patients. The nodal detection rate was 98.7% for ICG vs. 97.5% for Tc, confirming the non-inferiority of ICG. All metastatic SLNs were identified by both methods [37]. A meta-analysis in breast cancer patients compared the diagnostic accuracy of blue dye and Tc with ICG. ICG was found to be superior to blue dye in terms of detection rate of patients and SLNs, as well as the FNR. ICG was furthermore significantly superior to Tc regarding the detection rate of patients, SLNs, positive SLNs and the FNR. When comparing ICG with the combined blue dye and

Tc technique, no significant differences were found [38]. Another meta-analysis in breast cancer patients confirmed these findings, showing a higher identification rate for SLNs and a significantly higher identification rate for metastatic SLNs with ICG as compared to conventional tracers [39]. A recent systematic review and meta-analysis demonstrated that ICG might be a non-inferior alternative to Tc for intraoperative guidance in SLNB of cutaneous melanoma. While Tc identified a significantly higher number of SLNs and metastatic SLNs in prospective studies, no significant differences were found concerning the identification of metastatic patients or the FNR [20]. In endometrial and cervical cancer, ICG has already become the tracer of choice to perform SLNB due to its superior diagnostic accuracy [44]. In patients with vulvar cancer, a combination of ICG and Tc resulted in a better detection rate than the standard combination of blue dye and Tc [45].

2.4 Hybrid tracers

As both Tc and ICG have their limitations and drawbacks, these two approaches are sometimes combined in clinical practice, using both methods independent from one another. However, there has also been the idea of directly combining the two contrast agents. In 2009, a hybrid tracer was developed that linked ICG and Tc on a molecular level in an effort to harvest the above-mentioned benefits of both tracers in a single agent [25], which is injected 18 to 24 hours before the surgery [46].

The hybrid approach improves optical guidance compared to blue dye, especially in complex anatomical regions such as the head and neck and pelvic basins. Furthermore, hybrid tracers have been shown to facilitate the excision of SLNs located near the injection site as, unlike free ICG, no leakage of hybrid tracer into surrounding tissue was observed. Finally, no adverse events have been reported [47]. Because ICG assumes the lymphatic migratory characteristics of Tc, it also has a significantly longer retention period in SLNs than free ICG, ensuring the excision of SLNs only [25]. On the other hand, in SLNs located deeper than 1 cm or for patients with a higher BMI, surgeons rely on radioactive signaling [47]. Thus, hybrid tracers combine the advantages of two successful techniques to allow for an improved SLNB.

The superiority of this technique compared to the standard combination of blue dye and Tc has been shown in various malignancies including skin, oral cavity, penile, prostate and vulvar cancer. Kleinjan et al. identified 99% of SLNs by gamma tracing and 95% by fluorescence. The hybrid tracer had a significantly higher accuracy than blue dye. The concomitant use of blue dye did not improve prognosis or recurrence-free survival. The combined FNR of all malignancies was 14% and specific FNR were in line with previous literature [47]. In a systematic review and meta-analysis of head and neck malignancies, the hybrid tracer technique was found to be significantly superior to ICG- or Tc-only approaches in detecting SLNs [25].

The technical challenges of producing the hybrid tracer and the associated higher costs resulting from this combination present the most limiting factor for its widespread introduction in clinical practice.

While the combination of Tc and ICG, as two tracers or as one hybrid tracer, leads to promising results regarding accuracy and combines their respective advantages as mentioned above, several new methods for lymphatic imaging for SLNB have also been explored in the recent past, including carbon nanoparticles, contrast-enhanced ultrasound, multispectral optoacoustic tomographic imaging, and superparamagnetic iron oxide nanoparticles. These are more niche approaches that, despite demonstrating very promising early results and being in use clinically in a few centers, mainly remain in an experimental phase and have not yet been adopted on a wider scale.

2.5 Carbon nanoparticles

Carbon nanoparticles (CNPs) are increasingly being investigated, mainly in gynecological cancer research. With a diameter of 150 nm, CNPs selectively enter lymphatic vessels and accumulate in SLNs. For instance, in endometrial cancer, 25 mg/ml and a total of 2 ml of sterile water solution of CNPs is injected at 3 and 9 o'clock of the cervix deeply (1 cm) and superficially (1–3 mm). After 20 minutes, the dissection begins. Once the anatomical region is incised, black-stained SLNs can be seen by eye under natural light without the need for any special equipment [48].

CNPs avoid preoperative injections, as necessary in LS [49], and accumulate in SLNs over a long time without leaking into adjacent tissues, contrary to blue dye [50]. CNPs have a diameter, allowing for selective passage and coloration in lymphatic vessels only. Its incapacity of entering blood vessels is given as the reason for avoiding adverse systemic events [50]. Studies in breast cancer and cervical cancer patients have indeed shown that CNPs did not result in any adverse events [49, 51]. In locations without the expensive LS or NIRFI equipment, CNPs might be a viable alternative.

Nevertheless, CNPs are also significantly limited by the fact that they rely on visual identification alone. Despite their intense color, tissue penetration is low and deep SLNs may be missed. Consequently, a higher BMI has also been associated with decreased detection rates [49]. Additionally, the lymph node basin must be obvious or assumed preoperatively, resulting in missed SLNs in cases of complex or unusual drainage patterns.

In breast cancer patients, CNPs were found to have a detection rate of 100% and a FNR of 11.1%, both superior results compared to the blue dye technique [51]. In cervical cancer, CNPs have a reported detection rate of 93.3% with a FNR of 0% [49].

2.6 Contrast-enhanced ultrasound

While ultrasound is the most common technique for preoperative evaluation of the lymph node status, its conventional technique cannot identify SLNs or sufficiently evaluate potential malignant characteristics. Contrast-enhanced Ultrasound (CEUS) was described by Sever et al. for identifying axillary SLNs in breast cancer patients. Gas-filled microbubbles were used as a contrast medium injected intradermally around the areola. Ultrasound was then used to visualize lymphatic channels and locate the SLN [52]. CEUS contrast media used today consists of gas-filled microbubbles suspended in a liquid. These microbubbles resonate when exposed to ultrasound waves. For instance, Perflutren contains octafluoropropane gas, whereas SonoVue contains sulfur hexafluoride gas [53]. The preferred method of administering the contrast media in breast cancer patients is an intradermal or subcutaneous injection around the areola, followed by the injection around the tumor [54]. 0.2–0.4 ml of contrast medium are administered depending on body weight. Gentle massage can be applied to stimulate lymph flow. Contrast pulse sequence ultrasound visualizes lymphatic channels. The lymph node first reached by the microbubbles is considered the SLN and presents areas of contrast medium accumulation. The SLN is morphologically assessed at 2, 4 and 6 minutes after injection and blue dye can be injected transcutaneously into the area of accumulation to mark its location [53, 55]. Other methods of marking the SLN preoperatively include skin marking, wire marking, and iodine-125 seed localization [56]. General signs for malignant SLNs during ultrasound include the absence of echogenic hilus, round shape, peripheral capsular vascularity or focal cortical thickening [57]. Specific criteria for malignant SLNs during CEUS, while difficult to establish, include early, heterogenous or absent, and hyperdense enhancement [53]. Furthermore, the time-intensity curve analysis quantifies several parameters of blood perfusion, including peak intensity, time to peak, rise time, mean passage time, wash-in slope and rise slope. A short rise time and time to peak, and increased peak intensity would be typical in malignant lesions [54].

Advantages of this technique include a quick and real-time visualization and the potential for carrying out a core-needle biopsy before surgical SLNB to assess the pathological status. CEUS-guided core-needle biopsy identifies metastases in more than half of patients with normal preoperative ultrasound [56]. Therefore, it might reduce surgical trauma and complications by preoperatively identifying patients who will need SLNB and those who will be able to avoid it as the metastasis is already histologically confirmed. Thus, it could also allow for an outpatient clinic approach in more patients, thereby reducing costs and healthcare overload. However, concerns about tumor seeding mentioned above remain. The examination takes on average around 19 minutes and is associated with a very steep learning curve [55]. No adverse events have been noted so far [58].

Of course, there are also some disadvantages to CEUS. Higher stage cancer or discontinuous lymphatic channels could result in missing a SLN [59]. Indeed, authors have shown that previous breast surgery or tumor cells blocking lymphatic vessels and nodes might prevent the contrast medium from accumulating in SLNs [60]. Furthermore, ultrasound methods are always operator-dependent [61]. Finally, CEUS has also been reported to identify a lower number of SLNs compared to standard techniques [55].

A systematic review and meta-analysis examining the diagnostic accuracy of CEUS-guided SLNB in breast cancer found a preoperative localization rate for SLNs of 70–100%. Interestingly, the authors found a significantly higher risk of metastasis in SLNs identified by CEUS compared to those not identified by CEUS, possibly indicating a more accurate selection of SLNs. In the meta-analysis, a sensitivity of 98% and specificity of 100% of SLN metastases were found. To be noted, the included studies presented a variety of contrast agents, injection techniques, combined localization methods and SLN marking used [62]. Other studies found a sensitivity and specificity of 75% and 100% [55], or 91% and 86% [63], respectively, each in breast cancer patients. Wang et al. compared blue dye-combined CEUS with a blue dye-only approach. The combined approach had a higher identification rate than the blue dye-only approach. No significant difference was found for recurrence-free survival between the two groups, with the false-negative rate for CEUS being at 30.8% after a median follow-up of 50 months [64]. Research about SLN detection with CEUS is largely restricted to breast cancer patients. Few studies have evaluated its accuracy in other malignancies. In patients with vulvar cancer, inguinal CEUS with SLN identification and wire marking was performed and resulted in a sensitivity of 81.2% for identifying inguinal SLNs compared to standard techniques, while all metastatic SLNs identified by standard techniques were also identified by CEUS [65]. In patients with head and neck malignancies, detection was successful in 80% of cases with a correct prediction of metastatic status in 87.5% [66]. In a melanoma swine model using Sonazoid (perflubutane), 67% of SLNs identified by CEUS contained metastases, compared to only 44% of those detected by the control blue dye. However, all SLNs identified by CEUS were also identified by blue dye [67].

2.7 Multispectral optoacoustic tomographic imaging

Multispectral optoacoustic tomographic imaging (MSOT) is a recent technique that uses a probe to detect ultrasonic waves generated by thermoelastic expansion resulting from laser-induced emission. Colloidal nanobeacons and ICG have been proposed as contrast media because of their accumulation in the first lymph node and return of a signal with optimal signal-to-noise ratio. Its technique has found a special application in melanoma SLNB because of the special properties of cancer cell melanin, which may serve as a natural contrast agent [17]. The idea is to inject ICG peritumorally and to observe the lymphatic drainage in real-time with two-dimensional MSOT imaging before incision. After localization of the SLN, the incision is made and the SLN is further localized through fluorescence imaging (NIRFI) until the excision. In their pioneering study, Stoffels et al. used a handheld MSOT system (Acuity Echo, iThera Medical GmbH). Nanosecond excitation laser pulses with six wavelengths between 700 and 900 nm and a 256-element detector array provided cross-sectional images with a 4 × 4 cm^2 field of view. The emitted optoacoustic signals were tomographically reconstructed. In order to separate individual absorbers, multispectral illumination was used at the mentioned wavelengths. The authors used spectral unmixing in order to increase the spatial detection sensitivity of ICG [68].

MSOT offers very high spatial and temporal resolution [17]. As discussed above, the widespread introduction of ICG-based NIRFI in clinical practice has been limited by insufficient penetration depths, a disadvantage that might be overcome by MSOT. Especially when combined with ultrasonography for image correlation as well as morphological and anatomical information, transcutaneous identification of SLN basins was successful [68]. Indeed, authors have shown that MSOT of ICG-labeled SLNs reliably identifies SLNs with a penetration depth of up to 5 cm [69], which would be particularly relevant in the case of axillary SLNs. Again, no adverse events were reported in published studies [68]. The method allows real-time imaging and would avoid the need for a radioactive tracer, shortening inpatient hospital stays and thereby reducing healthcare costs. Its main disadvantage is the sparse literature on this method, with only two studies examining SLN identification with MSOT, both of them restricted to melanoma [68, 69]. This entails an insecurity as for the results of these studies. Furthermore, its low specificity, operator-dependent results and lack of availability have been pointed out [17].

In the rare studies evaluating its diagnostic accuracy, MSOT seems to be a promising method for SLN identification. Previous authors have compared the diagnostic accuracy of MSOT and ICG-based NIRFI to LS and SPECT-CT. Preoperative MSOT/ICG identified 94.6% of SLN basins identified by LS/SPECT-CT. To be noted, the authors combined MSOT with an integrated, pulse-echo ultrasonography, which allowed further improvement of SLN basin identification from 76.4% to 94.6% of basins identified by LS/SPECT-CT. Intraoperatively, 96.4% of Tc-labeled SLNs identified by gamma-probe were also identified by MSOT and following NIRFI. No positive SLN was missed by MSOT, resulting in a FNR of 0% for a mean follow-up of 26.7 months. The authors concluded that MSOT with ICG was not inferior to Tc-based LS in all anatomical regions [68].

2.8 Superparamagnetic iron oxide nanoparticles

Magnetic tracing options and superparamagnetic iron oxide nanoparticles (SPION) are yet another option that has been increasingly investigated. After injection, these particles accumulate in macrophages of normal lymph nodes, leading to a signal loss. Neoplastic areas of the node, on the other hand, stand out due to persistent signaling on imaging or magnetic probes [17]. The technique itself consists in injecting 2 ml of the magnetic tracer called Sienna+ and 3 ml of saline solution perilesionally. Sienna+ consists of SPION coated with carboxydextran. After 20 minutes, a handheld Sentimag magnetometer is used to localize the marker in the lymph node basins. The Sentimag probe creates an alternating magnetic field which magnetizes the nanoparticles. These are then detected by the probe. The probe produces a sound and signals proportionally to the intensity of the magnetic field. Following the signal strength, an incision is made and the handheld probe continues to be used until the SLN is identified. Additionally, SLNs may be discolored brown by the tracer. Similarly to the standard Tc technique, this is continued until the remaining tissue has a signal of less than 10% of the hottest SLN identified [70].

Advantages when compared to Tc-based LS include avoidance of radiation exposure. Furthermore, execution time is shorter, and nuclear medicine departments are not required to do so. Its technique combines visual guidance by brown discoloration and acoustic guidance with a handheld probe in one single tracer. Finally, Sienna+ can be used as a contrast medium in MRI imagery. A preoperative MRI with inhomogeneous uptake of the contrast medium in SLNs might replace preoperative LS for the identification of affected basins [70]. SPION-based MRI also has a higher resolution than Tc-based LS and identifies even small SLNs, allowing for the differentiation of several SLNs close to one another. This is particularly helpful in pelvic SLNB of prostate cancer patients [71].

On the other hand, it cannot be used in patients with hemosiderosis because of the risk of iron overload disease, hypersensitivity to dextran compounds [72], or presenting pacemakers or metal implants [39]. In overweight or elderly patients, the uptake of the magnetic tracer may take more time intraoperatively [70]. Importantly, residual SPION after SLNB may create void artifacts on follow-up MRI imaging for up to 3.6 years after the operation. This may however be avoided with the use of low-dose SPION injections [73]. The technique is furthermore associated with skin staining [74]. Other disadvantages include the need for plastic, non-magnetic surgical instruments to avoid signal interferences, which is especially difficult during laparoscopic interventions. Also, the Sentimag probe only reaches a penetration depth of around 2 cm, which might pose problems in axillary dissection or adipose patients, especially [71]. Indeed, patients who underwent SPION-based axillary SLNB had lower identification rates than those with groin SLNB in previous studies [74]. Finally, the magnetometer diameter is larger than that of the gamma probes, necessitating frequent rebalancing of the probe [39].

Previous authors have compared the magnetic Sentimag technique with radioactive tracing in breast cancer patients and found an SLN detection rate of 88.9% for radioactive and 89.5% for magnetic tracing [70]. The magnetic technique was non-inferior to the standard LS technique, with an identification rate of 95% for standard and 94.4% for magnetic technique in another breast cancer study [72]. Similarly, in prostate cancer, a SLN detection rate of 100% has been reported with a specificity of 97% and a FNR of 0% when compared to extended lymph node dissection [71]. The MELAMAG trial compared the SPION technique with the standard technique of blue dye and Tc in melanoma patients. SLN identification rate with the standard technique was 97.7%, while it was 95.3% with the magnetic technique. While these results were promising, it did not reach the predefined non-inferiority margin in this study [74]. SPION have also been combined with ICG as a magnetic fluorescent hybrid tracer in prostate cancer patients, resulting in improved SLN identification [75].

3. Conclusions

SLNB is an essential step in staging and treatment of patients suffering from a variety of malignant tumors. The last decades have seen increasingly precise technical approaches to visualizing specific lymph nodes in their basins, while surgeons have optimized the procedure of SLNB. A reliable and accurate method for preoperative planning as well as intraoperative, real-time guidance and confirmation of the SLN, is indispensable during this surgery.

While Tc-based LS remains the current standard of care in SLNB, authors have searched for alternatives due to the important disadvantages that come with this technique. These alternatives have in part been shown to equal the diagnostic accuracy of LS in several malignancies or to improve it in a singular or combined approach. The advantages and disadvantages of these techniques differ significantly and the success of their application depends on the type of cancer, anatomical location of SLNs, patient characteristics and several other factors. Future studies and changes in health-economic considerations will determine if one of these techniques can replace LS as the standard of care. However, rather than a single method it seems more likely that a combined approach taking into account specific tumor and patient characteristics will emerge as the best option. This optimal approach should come with minimal side effects and improved patient experience, while maintaining diagnostic accuracy and oncologic safety.

Acknowledgements

No funding was received.

Conflict of interest

The authors declare no conflict of interest.

Author details

Marcus Wölffer and Cédric Zubler*
Department of Plastic and Hand Surgery, Inselspital University Hospital Bern, University of Bern, Bern, Switzerland

*Address all correspondence to: cedric.zubler@unibe.ch

References

[1] Morton DL, Wen DR, Wong JH, Economou JS, Cagle LA, Storm FK, et al. Technical details of intraoperative lymphatic mapping for early stage melanoma. Archives of Surgery. 1992;**127**(4):392-399

[2] Moncayo VM, Grady EE, Alazraki NP, Aarsvold JN. Sentinel-lymph-node multicenter trials. Seminars in Nuclear Medicine. 2020;**50**(1):56-74

[3] Morrison S, Han D. Re-evaluation of sentinel lymph node biopsy for melanoma. Current Treatment Options in Oncology. 2021;**22**(3):22

[4] Gershenwald JE, Scolyer RA, Hess KR, Sondak VK, Long GV, Ross MI, et al. Melanoma staging: Evidence-based changes in the American Joint Committee on Cancer eighth edition cancer staging manual. CA: A Cancer Journal for Clinicians. 2017;**67**(6):472-492

[5] Crystal JS, Thompson JF, Hyngstrom J, Caracò C, Zager JS, Jahkola T, et al. Therapeutic value of sentinel lymph node biopsy in patients with melanoma: A randomized clinical trial. JAMA Surgery. 2022;**157**(9):835-842

[6] Faries MB, Thompson JF, Cochran AJ, Andtbacka RH, Mozzillo N, Zager JS, et al. Completion dissection or observation for sentinel-node metastasis in melanoma. The New England Journal of Medicine. 2017;**376**(23):2211-2222

[7] Wu CE, Hsieh CH, Chang CJ, Yeh JT, Kuo TT, Yang CH, et al. Prognostic factors for Taiwanese patients with cutaneous melanoma undergoing sentinel lymph node biopsy. Journal of the Formosan Medical Association. 2015;**114**(5):415-421

[8] Long GV, Menzies AM, Scolyer RA. Neoadjuvant checkpoint immunotherapy and melanoma: The time is now. Journal of Clinical Oncology. 2023;**41**(17):3236-3248

[9] Eigentler TK, Hoge J, Garbe C, Schadendorf D, et al. S3 – Leitlinie zur Diagnostik, Therapie und Nachsorge des Melanom. Journal der Deutschen Dermatologischen Gesellschaft. 2020;**18**(10):1079-1208

[10] Astvatsaturyan K, Ramazyan A, Bose S. Is ultrasound-guided fine needle aspiration biopsy of axillary lymph nodes a viable alternative to sentinel lymph node biopsy? Diagnostic Cytopathology. 2021;**49**(10):1099-1109

[11] Kadan Y, Baron A, Brezinov Y, Ben Arie A, Fishman A, Beiner M. Predictors of uncommon location of sentinel nodes in endometrial and cervical cancers. Gynecologic Oncology Reports. 2022;**39**:100917

[12] Sumner WE 3rd, Ross MI, Mansfield PF, Lee JE, Prieto VG, Schacherer CW, et al. Implications of lymphatic drainage to unusual sentinel lymph node sites in patients with primary cutaneous melanoma. Cancer. 2002;**95**(2):354-360

[13] Stewart CL, Gleisner A, Kwak J, Chapman B, Pearlman N, Gajdos C, et al. Implications of sentinel lymph node drainage to multiple basins in head and neck melanoma. Annals of Surgical Oncology. 2017;**24**(5):1386-1391

[14] Li X, Chen S, Duan Y, Guo H, Jiang L, Kong X, et al. Identification and preservation of stained non-sentinel lymph nodes in breast cancer. Oncology Letters. 2020;**20**(6):373

[15] Wong SL, Balch CM, Hurley P, Agarwala SS, Akhurst TJ, Cochran A, et al. Sentinel lymph node biopsy for melanoma: American Society of Clinical Oncology and Society of Surgical Oncology joint clinical practice guideline. Journal of Clinical Oncology. 2012;**30**(23):2912-2918

[16] Moncayo VM, Aarsvold JN, Alazraki NP. Lymphoscintigraphy and sentinel nodes. Journal of Nuclear Medicine. 2015;**56**(6):901-907

[17] Cuccurullo V, Rapa M, Catalfamo B, Cascini GL. Role of nuclear sentinel lymph node mapping compared to new alternative imaging methods. Journal of Personalized Medicine. 2023;**13**(8):1219

[18] Mariani G, Erba P, Manca G, Villa G, Gipponi M, Boni G, et al. Radioguided sentinel lymph node biopsy in patients with malignant cutaneous melanoma: The nuclear medicine contribution. Journal of Surgical Oncology. 2004;**85**(3):141-151

[19] Peek MC, Charalampoudis P, Anninga B, Baker R, Douek M. Blue dye for identification of sentinel nodes in breast cancer and malignant melanoma: A systematic review and meta-analysis. Future Oncology. 2017;**13**(5):455-467

[20] Wölffer M, Liechti R, Constantinescu M, Lese I, Zubler C. Sentinel lymph node detection in cutaneous melanoma using indocyanine green-based near-infrared fluorescence imaging: A systematic review and meta-analysis. Cancers (Basel). 2024;**16**(14):2523

[21] Tokin CA, Cope FO, Metz WL, Blue MS, Potter BM, Abbruzzese BC, et al. The efficacy of Tilmanocept in sentinel lymph mode mapping and identification in breast cancer patients: A comparative review and meta-analysis of the ^{99}mTc-labeled nanocolloid human serum albumin standard of care. Clinical & Experimental Metastasis. 2012;**29**(7):681-686

[22] Cattin F, Fogacci T, Frisoni GB, Fabiocchi L, Dellachiesa L, Semprini G, et al. Icg versus 99tc in breast surgery-how to match quality health care and costs reduction: A cost effectiveness study. Journal of Cancer Science and Therapy. 2017;**9**:340-342

[23] Lützen U, Naumann CM, Dischinger J, Marx M, Baumann R, Zhao Y, et al. 10-year experience regarding the reliability and morbidity of radio guided lymph node biopsy in penile cancer patients and the associated radiation exposure of medical staff in this procedure. BMC Urology. 2016;**16**(1):47

[24] Valiveru RC, Agarwal G, Agrawal V, Gambhir S, Mayilvaganan S, Chand G, et al. Low-cost fluorescein as an alternative to radio-colloid for sentinel lymph node biopsy—A prospective validation study in early breast cancer. World Journal of Surgery. 2020;**44**(10):3417-3422

[25] Wang B, Ma X, Zhang X, Zhang X, Guan S, Xiao T, et al. Application value of a hybrid tracer during sentinel lymph node biopsy for head and neck malignancies: A systematic review and meta-analysis. European Journal of Surgical Oncology. 2024;**50**(6):108340

[26] Whitman GJ, AlHalawani RH, Karbasian N, Krishnamurthy R. Sentinel lymph node evaluation: What the radiologist needs to know. Diagnostics (Basel). 2019;**9**(1):12

[27] Manca G, Romanini A, Rubello D, Mazzarri S, Boni G, Chiacchio S, et al. A critical reappraisal of false negative sentinel lymph node biopsy in melanoma. The Quarterly Journal

of Nuclear Medicine and Molecular Imaging. 2014;**58**(2):105-113

[28] Wang L, Liu S, Xu T, Yuan L, Yang X. Sentinel lymph node mapping in early-stage cervical cancer: Meta-analysis. Medicine (Baltimore). 2021;**100**(34):e27035

[29] Doepker MP, Yamamoto M, Applebaum MA, Patel NU, Jaime Montilla-Soler M, Sarnaik AA, et al. Comparison of single-photon emission computed tomography-computed tomography (SPECT/CT) and conventional planar lymphoscintigraphy for sentinel node localization in patients with cutaneous malignancies. Annals of Surgical Oncology. 2017;**24**(2):355-361

[30] Luan T, Li Y, Wu Q, Wang Y, Huo Z, Wang X, et al. Value of quantitative SPECT/CT lymphoscintigraphy in improving sentinel lymph node biopsy in breast cancer. The Breast Journal. 2022;**2022**:6483318

[31] Stoffels I, Boy C, Pöppel T, Kuhn J, Klötgen K, Dissemond J, et al. Association between sentinel lymph node excision with or without preoperative SPECT/CT and metastatic node detection and disease-free survival in melanoma. Journal of the American Medical Association. 2012;**308**(10):1007-1014

[32] Chapman BC, Gleisner A, Kwak JJ, Hosokawa P, Paniccia A, Merkow JS, et al. SPECT/CT improves detection of metastatic sentinel lymph nodes in patients with head and neck melanoma. Annals of Surgical Oncology. 2016;**23**(8):2652-2657

[33] Benke M, Wocial K, Lewandowska W, Rutkowski P, Teterycz P, Jarek P, et al. Value of planar lymphoscintigraphy (PL) versus SPECT/CT in evaluation of sentinel lymph node in trunk melanoma - one center, large series retrospective study. Nuclear Medicine Review. Central & Eastern Europe. 2018;**21**(2):79-84

[34] Tardelli E, Mazzarri S, Rubello D, Gennaro M, Fantechi L, Duce V, et al. Sentinel lymph node biopsy in cutaneous melanoma: Standard and new technical procedures and clinical advances. A systematic review of the literature. Clinical Nuclear Medicine. 2016;**41**(12):e498-e507

[35] Argentou MI, Iliopoulos E, Verras GI, Mulita F, Tchabashvili L, Spyridonidis T, et al. Study on intraoperative localization of sentinel lymph nodes using freehand SPECT in breast cancer patients. Wideochirurgia i Inne Techniki Małoinwazyjne. 2022;**17**(4):641-651

[36] Vahabzadeh-Hagh AM, Blackwell KE, Abemayor E, St John MA. Sentinel lymph node biopsy in cutaneous melanoma of the head and neck using the indocyanine green SPY elite system. American Journal of Otolaryngology. 2018;**39**(5):485-488

[37] Dumitru D, Ghanakumar S, Provenzano E, Benson JR. A prospective study evaluating the accuracy of indocyanine green (ICG) fluorescence compared with radioisotope for sentinel lymph node (SLN) detection in early breast cancer. Annals of Surgical Oncology. 2022;**29**(5):3014-3020

[38] Yin R, Ding LY, Wei QZ, Zhou Y, Tang GY, Zhu X. Comparisons of ICG-fluorescence with conventional tracers in sentinel lymph node biopsy for patients with early-stage breast cancer: A meta-analysis. Oncology Letters. 2021;**21**(2):114

[39] Rocco N, Velotti N, Pontillo M, Vitiello A, Berardi G, Accurso A, et al. New techniques versus standard mapping for sentinel lymph node biopsy in breast cancer: A systematic review

and meta-analysis. Updates in Surgery. 2023;**75**(6):1699-1710

[40] Gilmore DM, Khullar OV, Gioux S, Stockdale A, Frangioni JV, Colson YL, et al. Effective low-dose escalation of indocyanine green for near-infrared fluorescent sentinel lymph node mapping in melanoma. Annals of Surgical Oncology. 2013;**20**(7):2357-2363

[41] Murawa D, Hirche C, Dresel S, Hünerbein M. Sentinel lymph node biopsy in breast cancer guided by indocyanine green fluorescence. The British Journal of Surgery. 2009;**96**(11):1289-1294

[42] Lese I, Constantinescu MA, Leckenby JI, Zubler C, Alberts I, Hunger RE, et al. Transcutaneous sentinel lymph node detection in cutaneous melanoma with indocyanine green and near-infrared fluorescence: A diagnostic sensitivity study. Medicine (Baltimore). 2022;**101**(36):e30424

[43] Namikawa K, Tsutsumida A, Tanaka R, Kato J, Yamazaki N. Limitation of indocyanine green fluorescence in identifying sentinel lymph node prior to skin incision in cutaneous melanoma. International Journal of Clinical Oncology. 2014;**19**(1):198-203

[44] Laufer J, Scasso S, Papadia A. Different tracers for sentinel node detection in gynecologic oncology. Current Opinion in Oncology. 2024;**36**(5):371-375

[45] Rundle S, Korompelis P, Ralte A, Bewick D, Ratnavelu N. A comparison of ICG-NIR with blue dye and technetium for the detection of sentinel lymph nodes in vulvar cancer. European Journal of Surgical Oncology. 2023;**49**(2):481-485

[46] Sánchez-Izquierdo N, Vidal-Sicart S, Campos F, Torné A, Angeles MA, Migliorelli F, et al. Detection of the sentinel lymph node with hybrid tracer (ICG-[(99m) Tc]Tc-albumin nanocolloid) in intermediate- and high-risk endometrial cancer: A feasibility study. EJNMMI Research. 2021;**11**(1):123

[47] Klein Jan GH, van Werkhoven E, van den Berg NS, Karakullukcu MB, Zijlmans H, van der Hage JA, et al. The best of both worlds: A hybrid approach for optimal pre- and intraoperative identification of sentinel lymph nodes. European Journal of Nuclear Medicine and Molecular Imaging. 2018;**45**(11):1915-1925

[48] He M, Liang S, Deng H, Zhang G, Wang Z, Yang X, et al. Comparing carbon nanoparticles and indocyanine green for sentinel lymph node mapping in endometrial cancer: A randomized-controlled single-center trial. Journal of Surgical Oncology. 2023;**128**(2):332-343

[49] Wang Y, Dan Z, Yuan G, Zhang G, Liu S, Zhang Y, et al. Detection of sentinel lymph node in laparoscopic surgery for uterine cervical cancer using carbon nanoparticles. Journal of Surgical Oncology. 2020;**122**(5):934-940

[50] Du J, Zhang Y, Ming J, Liu J, Zhong L, Liang Q, et al. Evaluation of the tracing effect of carbon nanoparticle and carbon nanoparticle-epirubicin suspension in axillary lymph node dissection for breast cancer treatment. World Journal of Surgical Oncology. 2016;**14**(1):164

[51] Wu X, Lin Q, Chen G, Lu J, Zeng Y, Chen X, et al. Sentinel lymph node detection using carbon nanoparticles in patients with early breast cancer. PLoS ONE. 2015;**10**(8):e0135714

[52] Sever AR, Mills P, Jones SE, Mali W, Jones PA. Sentinel node identification

using microbubbles and contrast-enhanced ultrasonography. Clinical Radiology. 2012;**67**(7):687-694

[53] Jain R, Khanna R, Verma A, Mishra SP, Meena RN, Khanna S, et al. Evaluation of axillary lymph nodes in breast cancer patients with clinically negative axilla using contrast enhanced ultrasonography. World Journal of Surgical Oncology. 2024;**22**(1):211

[54] Yang Q, Fu Y, Wang J, Yang H, Zhang X. Advantages of contrast-enhanced ultrasound in the localization and diagnostics of sentinel lymph nodes in breast cancer. Journal of Zhejiang University. Science. B. 2023;**24**(11):985-997

[55] Buonomo OC, Materazzo M, Pellicciaro M, Iafrate G, Ielpo B, Rizza S, et al. Contrast-enhanced ultrasound using intradermal microbubble sulfur hexafluoride for identification of sentinel lymph nodes during breast cancer surgery: A clinical trial. Anticancer Research. 2023;**43**(2):557-567

[56] Nielsen Moody A, Bull J, Culpan AM, Munyombwe T, Sharma N, Whitaker M, et al. Preoperative sentinel lymph node identification, biopsy and localisation using contrast enhanced ultrasound (CEUS) in patients with breast cancer: A systematic review and meta-analysis. Clinical Radiology. 2017;**72**(11):959-971

[57] Rubaltelli L, Beltrame V, Scagliori E, Bezzon E, Frigo AC, Rastrelli M, et al. Potential use of contrast-enhanced ultrasound (CEUS) in the detection of metastatic superficial lymph nodes in melanoma patients. Ultraschall in der Medizin. 2014;**35**(1):67-71

[58] Shimazu K, Ito T, Uji K, Miyake T, Aono T, Motomura K, et al. Identification of sentinel lymph nodes by contrast-enhanced ultrasonography with Sonazoid in patients with breast cancer: A feasibility study in three hospitals. Cancer Medicine. 2017;**6**(8):1915-1922

[59] Barentsz MW, Verkooijen HM, Pijnappel RM, Fernandez MA, van Diest PJ, van der Pol CC, et al. Sentinel lymph node localization with contrast-enhanced ultrasound and an I-125 seed: An ideal prospective development study. International Journal of Surgery. 2015;**14**:1-6

[60] Luo Y, Chen J, Feng L, Cao W, Wu H, Ma M, et al. Study on sentinel lymph node and its lymphatic drainage pattern of breast cancer by contrast-enhanced ultrasound. Journal of Ultrasound in Medicine. 2022;**41**(11):2727-2737

[61] Pistolese CA, Lamacchia F, Tosti D, Anemona L, Ricci F, Censi M, et al. Reducing the number of unnecessary percutaneous biopsies: The role of second opinion by expert breast center radiologists. Anticancer Research. 2020;**40**(2):939-950

[62] Cui Q, Dai L, Li J, Xue J. Accuracy of CEUS-guided sentinel lymph node biopsy in early-stage breast cancer: A study review and meta-analysis. World Journal of Surgical Oncology. 2020;**18**(1):112

[63] Liu X, Wang M, Wang Q, Zhang H. Diagnostic value of contrast-enhanced ultrasound for sentinel lymph node metastasis in breast cancer: An updated meta-analysis. Breast Cancer Research and Treatment. 2023;**202**(2):221-231

[64] Wang X, Tang L, Huang W, Cui Z, Hu D, Zhong Z, et al. The combination of contrast-enhanced ultrasonography with blue dye for sentinel lymph node detection in clinically negative node breast cancer. Archives of Gynecology and Obstetrics. 2021;**304**(6):1551-1559

[65] Lahtinen O, Eloranta M, Anttila M, Kärkkäinen H, Sironen R, Vanninen R, et al. Preoperative sentinel lymph node localization in vulvar cancer: Preliminary experience with inguinal intradermal contrast-enhanced ultrasound. European Radiology. 2018;**28**(5):2089-2095

[66] Wakisaka N, Endo K, Kitazawa T, Shimode Y, Kato K, Moriyama-Kita M, et al. Detection of sentinel lymph node using contrast-enhanced agent, Sonazoid(™), and evaluation of its metastasis with superb microvascular imaging in oral and oropharyngeal cancers: A preliminary clinical study. Acta Oto-Laryngologica. 2019;**139**(1):94-99

[67] Bertelsen C, King KG, Swanson M, Duddalwar V, Pepper JP. Contrast-enhanced ultrasound with perflubutane for sentinel lymph node mapping in cutaneous melanoma: A pilot study. The Laryngoscope. 2019;**129**(5):1117-1122

[68] Stoffels I, Jansen P, Petri M, Goerdt L, Brinker TJ, Griewank KG, et al. Assessment of nonradioactive multispectral optoacoustic tomographic imaging with conventional lymphoscintigraphic imaging for sentinel lymph node biopsy in melanoma. JAMA Network Open. 2019;**2**(8):e199020

[69] Stoffels I, Morscher S, Helfrich I, Hillen U, Leyh J, Burton NC, et al. Metastatic status of sentinel lymph nodes in melanoma determined noninvasively with multispectral optoacoustic imaging. Science Translational Medicine. 2015;**7**(317):317ra199

[70] Izzo P, De Intinis C, Sibio S, Basso L, Polistena A, Gabriele R, et al. Sentinel lymph node detection in breast Cancer: An innovative technique. Diagnostics (Basel). 2023;**13**(12):2030

[71] Winter A, Engels S, Goos P, Süykers MC, Gudenkauf S, Henke RP, et al. Accuracy of magnetometer-guided sentinel lymphadenectomy after intraprostatic injection of superparamagnetic iron oxide nanoparticles in prostate cancer: The SentiMag pro II study. Cancers (Basel). 2019;**12**(1):32

[72] Douek M, Klaase J, Monypenny I, Kothari A, Zechmeister K, Brown D, et al. Sentinel node biopsy using a magnetic tracer versus standard technique: The SentiMAG multicentre trial. Annals of Surgical Oncology. 2014;**21**(4):1237-1245

[73] Christenhusz A, Pouw JJ, Simonis FFJ, Douek M, Ahmed M, Klaase JM, et al. Breast MRI in patients after breast conserving surgery with sentinel node procedure using a superparamagnetic tracer. European Radiology Experimental. 2022;**6**(1):3

[74] Anninga B, White SH, Moncrieff M, Dziewulski P, Geh JLC, Klaase J, et al. Magnetic technique for sentinel lymph node biopsy in melanoma: The MELAMAG trial. Annals of Surgical Oncology. 2016;**23**(6):2070-2078

[75] Michalik B, Engels S, Otterbach MC, Frerichs J, Suhrhoff PE, van Oosterom MN, et al. A new bimodal approach for sentinel lymph node imaging in prostate cancer using a magnetic and fluorescent hybrid tracer. European Journal of Nuclear Medicine and Molecular Imaging. 2024;**51**(10):2922-2928

Chapter 3

Research Progress in Diagnosis and Treatment of Lymphorrhagia after Neck, Chest, and Abdominal Surgery

Yang Gao and Jianchun Cui

Abstract

Lymphatic leakage is a rare complication of neck, chest, and abdominal surgery. The occurrence of severe lymphatic leakage can lead to a series of serious consequences. For different degrees of lymphatic leakage, the treatment can be divided into conservative treatment and surgical treatment. For mild and moderate neck surgery and breast cancer axillary lymphorrhaphy, low-fat diet and locally effective compression are the key links of conservative treatment. Severe lymphatic leakage requires surgical treatment, and traditional surgical treatment is difficult, but modified lymphangiography through inguinal lymph node puncture or combined with thoracic catheter embolization has recently been proved to be effective, minimally invasive and safe.

Keywords: thoracic duct, lymphatic leakage, chylous fluid, lymphangiography, thoracic duct embolization

1. Introduction

The thoracic duct, also known as the left lymphatic duct, is formed by the confluence of the left and right lumbar trunk and intestinal trunk in front of the first to second lumbar vertebrae. The initial part is cystic enlargement, called chylocisterna. The thoracic duct receives the left trunk of the neck, the subclavian trunk, and the left bronchomediastinal trunk, and is then injected into the left venous horn, with a pair of valves at the entrance to prevent lymphatic reflux. There is generally no valve at the entrance of these three main trunks, which is one of the important factors for the metastasis of cancer cells from thoracic and abdominal tumors to the cervical root lymph nodes through the thoracic duct. The right lymphatic duct is a short trunk formed by the conjoining of the right cervical trunk, right subclavian trunk, and right bronchomediastinal trunk. This catheter collected lymph from the right upper limb, right head and neck, right lung, right heart, and right chest wall and injected it into the right subclavian vein (or right venous corner) (**Figure 1**). Chylous fluid is a kind of intestinal lymph fluid, which can produce 3–5 L per day, mainly composed of lymph fluid, immune cells, and

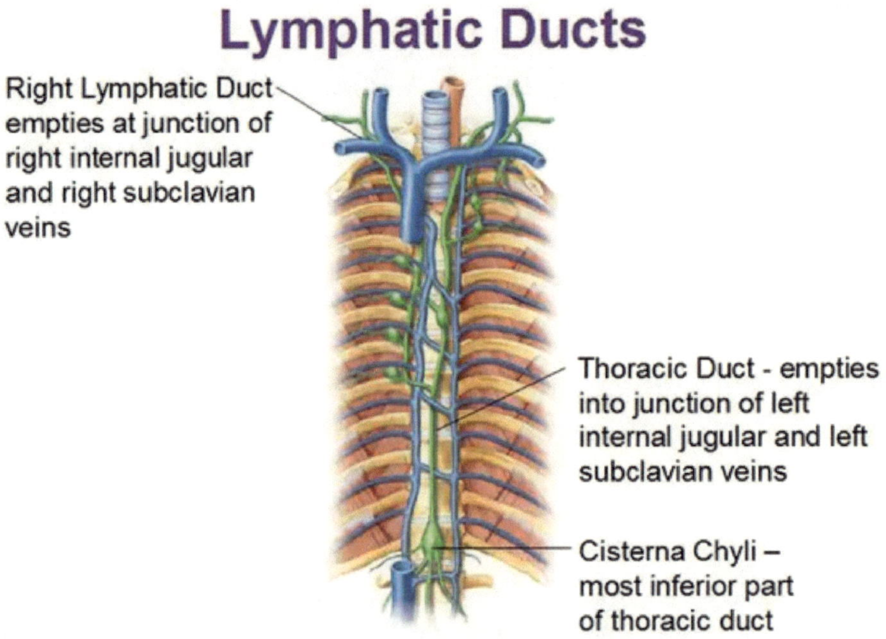

Figure 1.
Overview of lymphatic duct.

chylomicrons, and contains a lot of triglycerides. The chyle fluid is collected into the enteric lymphatic vessels through the mesenteric lymphatic vessels, then merges with the chyle fluid of the left and right lumbar lymphatic vessels into the chyle cisterna, and finally infuses into the left venous angle through the thoracic catheter, a process called chyle reflux [1]. If the thoracic duct breaks at different locations, it may lead to lymphatic leakage (chylous neck, chylous thorax, chylous abdomen).

Lymphatic leakage is a rare but serious complication of neck and chest operations, with an incidence of 2–8% [2], while the incidence of lymphorrhaphy in abdominal operations is relatively rare, with an incidence of about 0.26% [3]. Improper treatment of lymphatic leakage after neck surgery can lead to chyme accumulation, local flap floating, necrosis, and even fatal massive hemorrhage caused by exposure of neck arteries. Lymphatic leakage after axillary dissection of breast cancer can easily lead to subcutaneous fluid accumulation, affect the flap adhesion to the chest wall, and even cause flap necrosis, increasing the risk of infection. A large amount of chylous fluid leakage after thoracic and abdominal surgery can lead to the loss of a large amount of proteins, immune cells, lipids and other substances, resulting in water and electrolyte imbalance, malnutrition, reduced immunity, high risk of infection, poor surgical incision healing, and prolonged extubation and hospitalization of patients, increasing the incidence of postoperative infection and lower limb venous thrombosis [4]. It can also cause patients to fear the prognosis of the disease. It is very important to diagnose the lymphatic leakage of the neck, chest, and abdomen in the early stage and to use effective treatment. This chapter reviews the latest research progress in the diagnosis and treatment of postoperative lymphorrhagia in the neck, chest, and abdomen.

2. Causes of lymphatic leakage

Due to the anatomic variation of the thoracic duct in the neck, the end points of the thoracic duct can be located in the internal jugular vein, subclavian vein, external jugular vein, or even innominate vein. Moreover, the lymphatic duct wall is transparent and thin, which is often difficult to identify during operation. Lymphatic vessels are brittle and weak in resistance to tension, which are easy to be torn during operation. Lymphatic leakage after epigastric or retroperitoneal surgery may be caused by the absence of a large lymphatic output tube at the distal end of the lymph nodes in the removed area. Preoperative chemotherapy, low protein, and a large amount of ascites increase the risk of postoperative lymphorrhagia in patients with tumor. With the widespread use of ultrasonic knives, the risk of lymphatic leakage is also increasing due to the inaccuracy of ultrasonic knives in closing lymphatic vessels. In addition, the surgeon is not familiar with the anatomical structure, or chooses the surgical plan with large wounds, etc., which increases the risk of lymphatic leakage [5, 6].

3. Diagnosis of lymphatic leakage

Lymphatic leakage generally occurs 1–3 days after surgery, especially within 48 hours after eating. The clinical manifestations are increased drainage of the drainage tube, tasteless milky white drainage fluid, neck swelling, obvious feeling of trachea compression, and even dyspnea in patients with obstructed neck drainage. Unblocked axillary drainage can cause flaps in the armpit and chest wall. Unblocked drainage in the chest and abdomen can lead to persistent abdominal pain and distension, and even clinical manifestations such as nausea, vomiting, and hypoproteinemia. Internationally, lymphatic leakage is divided into light, medium, and severe according to the amount, the drainage flow of 50–200 ml/d is mild, 200–400 ml/d is moderate, and more than 400 ml/d is severe (**Figure 2**).

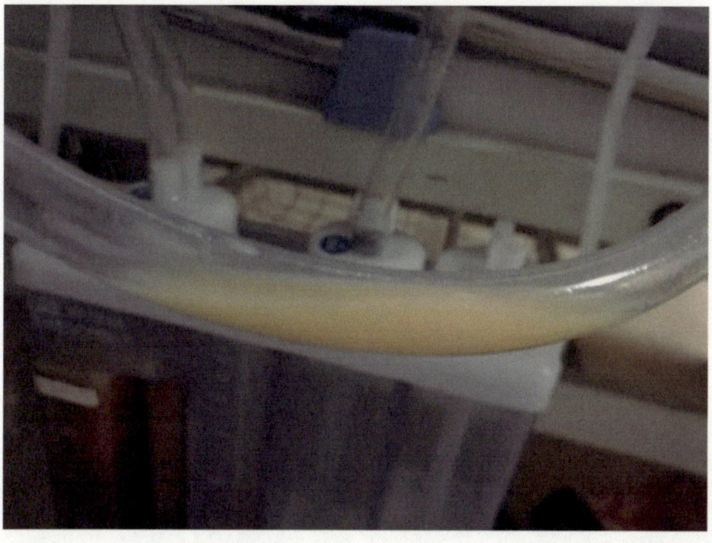

Figure 2.
Chylous fluid.

3.1 Laboratory diagnosis

The qualitative test of chylous of drainage fluid or puncture fluid is positive, or the triglyceride content of drainage fluid is >110 mg/dl(1.2 mmol/l), cholesterol concentration is <200 mmol/L, protein concentration is between 2.5 and 7 g/dl, glucose concentration is <100 mg/dl, and the cells are mainly lymphocytes [7], which can be diagnosed as lymphorrhea. In addition, the microscopic examination of chylomicron by drainage fluid and Sudan III staining also has suggestive effects.

3.2 Imaging diagnosis

Computed tomography (CT) and magnetic resonance imaging (MRI) are commonly used in clinical diagnosis of postoperative lymphatic leakage in the chest and abdomen, and can determine the location of lymphatic vessel damage. However, as the density of chylous fluid is similar to that of most pleural and abdominal effusions, it is difficult to distinguish it from other types of effusions, so CT and MRI have low diagnostic specificity for chylous pleural effusions and ascites [8].

Lymphangiography is the gold standard for clinical diagnosis of lymphangiography, including transnodal lymphangiography and ultrasound-guided intranodal lymphangiography. Compared with traditional dorsal foot lymphangiography, endonodal lymphangiography has the advantages of simplicity, less trauma, and shorter time, which has had a profound impact on the development of lymphangiography technology and lymphatic system interventional therapy. This technique is performed by direct puncture of the inguinal lymph nodes guided by a high-frequency (>7.5 MHz) ultrasonic probe, generally selecting a larger lymph node and placing the tip of the needle in the transition area between the cortex and the hilum of the lymph node, and then slowly injecting iodide at a rate of approximately 1 to 2 mL/5 min under intermittent fluoroscopy. The initial appearance is a small nodular stain, followed by the development of the associated branch lymphatic vessels, usually about 40 minutes after the initiation of iodide injection can be seen. In order to prevent the occurrence

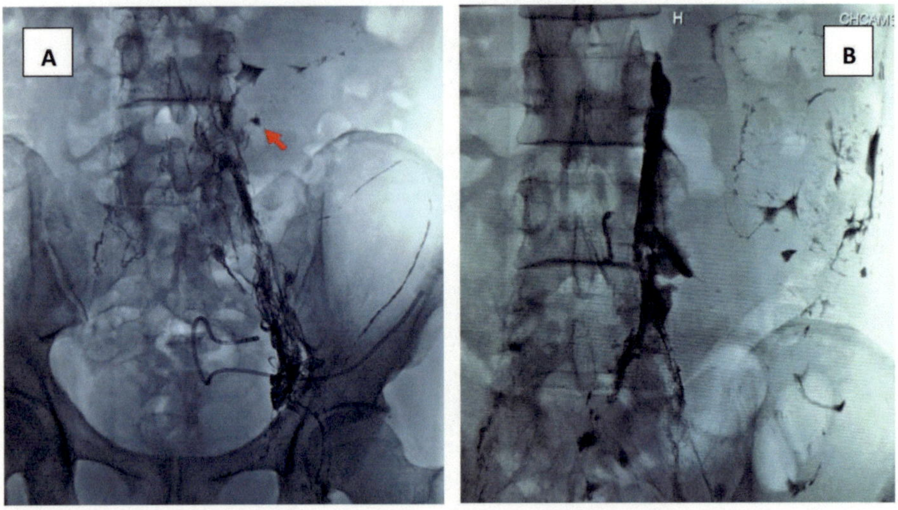

Figure 3.
A: lymphadenography found the rupture (red arrow); B: The rupture was completely sealed after embolization.

of pulmonary embolism, the amount of iodide on each side is generally not more than 10 mL (the total amount is not more than 20 mL). Lymphangiography not only has a clear diagnostic significance for lymphatic leakage, but also has certain therapeutic effects (**Figure 3**) [9].

Radionuclide lymphatic imaging is also a method to diagnose lymphatic leakage. This technique is to inject radionuclide 99mTc tracer subcutaneously or intradermal and then perform whole body imaging through single-photon emission-computed tomography (SPECT) to detect lymph flow and evaluate the tracer transport speed, lymph node distribution, number, and size. Identify defective lymphatic vessels [10]. But it is not widely used at present.

4. Treatment of lymphatic leakage

At present, the treatment of lymphatic leakage mainly includes conservative treatment and surgical treatment. Most mild and moderate lymphatic leakage can be cured by conservative treatment. If conservative treatment fails or the drainage exceeds 600 ml/d within 24 hours, especially if the drainage volume exceeds 2000 ml/d, surgical treatment is required [11, 12].

4.1 Conservative treatment

Psychotherapy: Lymphatic leakage, especially high-flow lymphatic leakage, can cause extreme fear of patients and their families, and patients should be timely and patiently psychological counseling to improve their confidence and sense of security.

Diet management: Once lymphorrhaphy is diagnosed, the normal diet should be changed to a low-fat diet. Normal diet contains a large number of lipids, which are the main components of chylous fluid. Dietary control can reduce the intake of lipids, reduce the production of chylous fluid, and promote lymphatic healing [13].

Local effective pressure dressing combined with vacuum suction is the key measure to treat lymphatic leakage after axillary dissection of neck and breast cancer. Clinical experiments have proved that local pressure bandaging combined with vacuum suction can effectively extract fluid leakage, make the flap close to the tissue, promote the adhesion of the wound to the surrounding tissue, eliminate the lacuna, close or narrow the leak, reduce the loss of lymph fluid, and completely close the leak when the local granulation tissue forms scars, thus healing lymphatic leakage [14, 15]. Traditional pressure dressing for cervical lymphorrhaphy mostly uses gauze to compress the supraclavicular fossa and the area near the trachea or the top of the armpit, and then fixes it with elastic bandages [16, 17], but the application is complicated and the effect is not obvious.

For cervical lymphatic leakage, external fixation of neck support and internal packing of cotton ball is the latest local pressure dressing method, which is simple and accurate. The key steps of this method are as follows: (1) Select a suitable neck support, and cut it appropriately to avoid the bone markers such as collarbone and mastoid, so as to prevent the skin from being damaged under pressure. (2) The packing of the cotton ball inside the neck support must be centered on the supraclavicular fossa and paratracheal to ensure that the compression position is accurate and does not shift. (3) Keep the vacuum negative pressure drainage smooth, closely observe the change of suction flow rate, there is no significant change in suction flow rate in 24 hours, and the position of cotton ball compression needs to be adjusted in time.

(4) Removal of drainage time: After the drainage flow was significantly reduced to less than 10 ml every 24 hours, the normal diet was changed for 3d, and the amount of drainage fluid remained unchanged; that is, the drainage tube was removed on the 14th day, and the neck ultrasound was re-examined 3 days after the drainage tube was removed to confirm that there was no recurrence of lymphatic leakage, so as to ensure complete clinical cure of lymphatic leakage [18]. This study emphasized the importance of low-fat diet, unblocked vacuum negative pressure drainage in the operative area, and effective local neck compression, which significantly shortened the length of hospital stay and reduced the cost of hospitalization (**Figure 4**).

Closed thoracic drainage may be used for conservative treatment of postoperative lymphatic leakage, and chemical pleuropexy may be performed during closed thoracic drainage to promote healing of the thoracic duct. Abdominal catheter drainage and abdominal compression bandaging are often used for postoperative lymphatic leakage, which can not only alleviate the clinical symptoms of patients, but also provide effective evidence for clinical evaluation of disease progression.

Intravenous medication: Some scholars recommend direct water fasting or even parenteral intravenous nutrition. Parenteral intravenous nutrition support, on the one hand, can correct nutrient consumption and metabolic dysfunction and reduce the generation of lymphatic leakage; on the other hand, promoting protein synthesis enhances plasma colloid osmotic pressure and promotes the absorption of accumulated fluid [19]. Some scholars have also suggested that somatostatin can inhibit the secretion of gastrointestinal and pancreatic peptide hormones, promote gastrointestinal peristalsis, and thus reduce lymphatic fluid production and intestinal absorption. However, it has the disadvantages of high cost and long treatment time.

Local injection of sclerotherapy: After the local extraction of chylous fluid, 50% glucose liquid, tetracycline, doxycycline, cell-bright, iodoform, or OK432 were injected to cause aseptic chemical inflammation, make the flap adhere to the wound, and promote the closure of lymphatic vessels, which is also one of the treatment methods [20, 21]. However, for patients treated with local injection of sclerosing agent, it is especially difficult to operate again after the recurrence of the original disease. Due to extensive local adhesion, normal surgical anatomic space will disappear, tissue inflammation and edema scar will be serious, and important surrounding structures such as internal jugular vein, recurrent laryngeal nerve, phrenic nerve, sympathetic nerve, and parathyroid gland will be easily damaged, leading to surgical

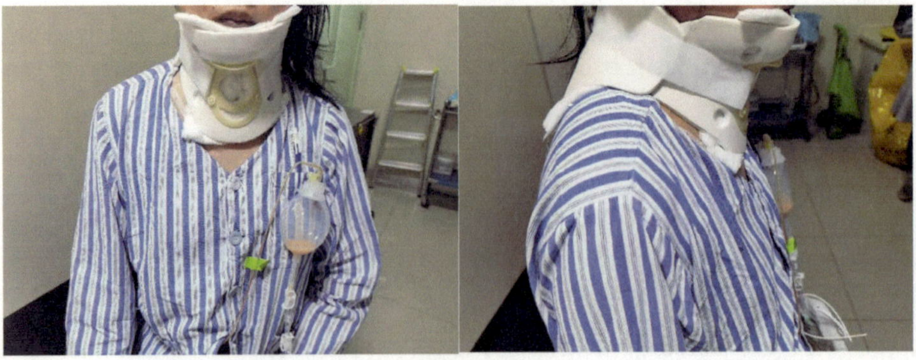

Figure 4.
External fixation of neck support combined with cotton ball packing in neck support.

failure. Therefore, local injection of sclerosing agent is generally used in cases where conservative treatment of lymphatic leakage is ineffective, and the risk of surgical treatment is greater.

4.2 Surgical treatment

Surgical treatment should be considered for patients with severe lymphatic leakage whose drainage volume persists for more than 5 days after conservative treatment or becomes ineffective after treatment for more than 2 weeks, or refractory nutritional or metabolic complications occur [22]. Traditional surgical treatment includes fistula ligation or suture, muscle flap filling, and covering.

Endoscopic lymphangiography or radionuclide lymphangiography is a commonly used surgical procedure. Lymphangiography or radionuclide lymphangiography is performed before surgery to locate the lymphatic leak. Damaged lymphatic vessels are repaired or lapped during surgery, and medical protein glue and gelatin sponge are sprayed on the wound. In patients with portal hypertension, transjugular intrahepatic portal vein shunt (TIPS) can be selected to reduce portal vein pressure, improve the status of abdominal lymphatic reflux, and facilitate the closure of lymphatic vessels. However, these operations will not only prolong the patient's hospital stay, but also aggravate the patient's condition and even lead to the death of the patient [13].

Recently, it has been reported in international literature that interventional surgery has made great progress in the study of diagnosis and treatment of lymphatic leakage, avoiding the severe lymphatic leakage patients undergoing more traumatic surgical operations. The combined application of spring coil and medical adhesive [23] is the most commonly used method for percutaneous thoracic catheter embolization.

The procedure is as follows: ① First, endonodal lymphangiography is performed to gradually develop the chylous cisterna and thoracic duct. ② Then, under fluoroscopy, 21 or 22G Chiba needle was used for percutaneous puncture of the chylous cisterna. The puncture point was generally located slightly to the right of the umbilical median line, avoiding adjacent structures such as aorta and right renal artery. In the process of puncture, the application of lateral fluoroscopy can help the puncture needle to enter the chylocisterna more accurately. The angle of the puncture needle should be slightly inclined to allow the subsequent guide wire to enter; after the needle enters the chylocisterna or larger lymphatic vessels, a 0.018 or 0.016 in microguide wire is used to enter the thoracic duct. ③ Then, after confirming that the position of the microguide wire in the thoracic catheter was safe and correct, 2 or 3F microcatheter was inserted, and a small amount of contrast agent was injected through the microcatheter to further determine the path of the thoracic catheter and the location and degree of leakage. ④ Finally, after catheterization of the thoracic catheter was performed and leakage was found, the micro-guide wire and micro-catheter were passed over the orifice of the fistula, and sufficient spring coils were placed near the orifice of the fistula to the ventral end to embolize the thoracic catheter. After the spring coils were placed, NBCA glue or Onyx glue were injected into the ventral end for further embolization to ensure complete embolization of the thoracic catheter. At present, percutaneous thoracic catheter embolization has been able to treat postoperative cervical lymphorrhagia, chylous pericardial effusion, chylothorax of newborn and chylomeric ascites, etc. [24]. Compared with traditional open surgery, lymphangiography combined with thoracic catheter embolization is more prominent in terms of minimally invasive, effective, and safe treatment of lymphorrhagia.

5. Conclusion

For patients with mild-to-moderate axillary lymph leakage from neck and breast cancer axillary dissection, adopting low-fat diet, vacuum negative pressure drainage, external fixation of neck support and accurate internal packing with cotton balls are the effective key links of conservative treatment. For patients with severe lymphatic leakage who have failed conservative treatment, endolymph node angiography combined with catheter embolization can be used, which is effective, minimally invasive and safe. The materials required for catheter embolization therapy are rare, which is one of the major bottlenecks in the development of this technique.

Author details

Yang Gao and Jianchun Cui*
Department of Thyroid and Breast Surgery, Liaoning Provincial People's Hospital, Shenyang, China

*Address all correspondence to: cjc7162003@aliyun.com

References

[1] Lv S, Wang Q, Zhao W, et al. A review of the postoperative lymphatic leakage. Oncotarget. 2017;**8**(40):69062-69075

[2] Itkin M, Nadolski GJ. Modern techniques of lymphangiography and interventions: Current status and future development. Cardiovascular and Interventional Radiology. 2018;**41**(3):366-376

[3] Delaney SW, Shi H, Shokrani A, et al. Management of Chyle leak after head and neck surgery: Review of current treatment strategies. International Journal of Otolaryngology. 2017;**2017**:8362874

[4] Zhang ZP, Xing ND. Influence factors of lymphatic leakage after laparoscopic radical cystectomy in 160 cases. Journal of Shandong University (Medical Edition). 2020;**58**(01):67-72

[5] McMullen C, Rorke D, Freeman J. Complications of bilateral neck dissection in thyroid cancer from a single high-volume center. JAMA Otolaryngology. Head & Neck Surgery. 2017;**14**(4):376-381

[6] Bin Z, Feng C, Lei Z. Causes and management of lymphatic leakage after cervical lymph node dissection for thyroid cancer: Clinical analysis of 20 cases. Journal of Trauma Surgery. 2019;**24**(1):143-145

[7] Chen L, Yu S, Chen S, et al. Application of imaging technique in thoracic duct anatomy. Ann Palliative Medicine. 2020;**9**(3):1249-1256

[8] Bhardwaj R, Vaziri H, Gautam A, et al. Chylous ascites: A review of pathogenesis, diagnosis and treatment. Journal of Clinical and Translational Hepatology. 2018;**6**(1):105-109

[9] Parmeggiani D, Gualtieri G, Terracciano G, et al. Prolonged iatrogenic thoracic duct chylous fistula in neck surgery: Conservative management or surgery? A literature review. Scandinavian Journal of Surgery. 2021;**110**(4):550-556

[10] Pappalardo M, Cheng MH. Lymphoscintigraphy for the diagnosis of extremity lymphedema: Current controversies regarding protocol, interpretation, and clinical application. Journal of Surgical Oncology. 2020;**121**(1):37-47

[11] Dorneden A, Olson G, 1, Nathan Boyd. Negative pressure wound therapy (wound VAC) in the treatment of chylous fistula after neck dissection. The Annals of Otology, Rhinology, and Laryngology. 2019;**128**(6):569-574

[12] Molena E, King E, Davies—Husband C. Octreotide versus oral dietary modification for the treatment of chylous fistula following neck dissection: A systematic review and meta-analysis. Clinical Otolaryngology. 2021;**46**(3):474-484

[13] Besselink MG, Van Rijssen LB, Bassi C, et al. Definition and classification of chyle leak after pancreatic operation: A consensus statement by the international study group on pancreatic surgery. Surgery. 2017;**161**(2):365-372

[14] Hao Weijing Y, Yang ZHENGX. Prevention and treatment of lymphatic leakage after central thyroid lymph node clearance. Chin Oncology. 2016;**43**(2):72-75. (in Chinese)

[15] Sun Tuan-QI W, Yi. The causes and prevention of lymphatic leakage during thyroid surgery. Chinese Journal of

Practical Surgery. 2012;**32**(5):372-374. (in Chinese)

[16] Chang GH, Lee CY, Tsai YT, et al. Strategic approach to massive chylous leakage after neck dissection. Healthcare (Basel). 2021;**9**(4):379

[17] Jianping L, Tao C, Yang W. Comprehensive treatment of severe lymphorrhagia after cervical dissection for thyroid cancer. Lingnan Modern Clinical Surgery. 2010;**10**(5):351-352

[18] Song R, Fei X, Cui J, Xuewei Y, Zhang Y, Li L, et al. Treatment strategy for chylous leakage after dissection of central lymph nodes in thyroid cancer. Annali Italiani di Chirurgia. 2020;**91**(6):692-696

[19] Baek Y, Won JH, Kong T-W, et al. Lymphatic leak occurring after surgical lymph node dissection: A preliminary study assessing the feasibility and outcome of lymphatic embolization. Cardio Vascular and Interventional Radiology. 2016;**39**(12):1728-1735

[20] Lee CW, Roh JL, Gong G, et al. Risk factors for recurrence of papillary thyroid carcinoma with clinically node-positive lateral neck. Annals of Surgical Oncology. 2015;**22**(1):117-124

[21] Kim SJ, Park SY, Lee YJ, et al. Risk factors for recurrence after therapeutic lateral neck dissection for primary papillary thyroid cancer. Annals of Surgical Oncology. 2014;**21**(6):1884-1890

[22] Kawasaki R, Sugimoto K, Fujii M, et al. Therapeutic effectiveness of diagnostic lymphangiography for refractory postoperative chylothorax and chylous ascites: Correlation with radiologic findings and preceding medical treatment. AJR. American Journal of Roentgenology. 2013;**201**(3):659-666

[23] Yammamoto M, Yamada K, Horikawa M, et al. Embolization of the thoracic duct by direct injection of n-butyl-2-cyanoacrylateglue via a puncture needle. Cardiovascular and Interventional Radiology. 2018;**41**(6):959-963

[24] Campisi CC, Boccardo F, Piazza C, et al. Evolution of chylous fistula management after neck dissection. Current Opinion in Otolaryngology and Head and Neck Surgery. 2013;**21**:150-156

Chapter 4

Bioengineering Lymphatic Vessels: A Novel Frontier in Regenerative Medicine

Jyothsna Butchireddy

Abstract

The lymphatic system is essential for sustaining fluid balance, lipid assimilation, and immune surveillance. Despite its significance, the lymphatic system has traditionally received less research attention than the cardiovascular system. Recent breakthroughs in bioengineering and regenerative medicine have created new possibilities for understanding and reconstructing lymphatic vessels. This chapter examines the most recent advancements in the bioengineering of lymphatic vessels, concentrating on the design, creation, and utilization of bioengineered lymphatic structures. We address the challenges and opportunities in this developing field, such as the integration of bioengineered lymphatic vessels with host tissues, the significance of biomaterials, and the prospects for clinical application. The chapter wraps up with a conversation about future pathways and the potential influence of bioengineered lymphatic vessels on addressing lymphatic disorders and advancing regenerative medicine.

Keywords: lymphatic vessels, bioengineering, regenerative medicine, biomaterials, tissue engineering

1. Introduction

The lymphatic system comprises a sophisticated network of vessels, nodes, and organs that is essential for preserving fluid homeostasis, immune activity, and lipid processing [1–5]. Malfunctions of the lymphatic system can result in various ailments, such as lymphedema, lymphangiectasia, and weakened immune responses [6]. Despite its important roles, the lymphatic system has garnered less focus within the realm of regenerative medicine than other organ systems [7]. Nevertheless, recent progress in bioengineering has begun to fill this void, presenting new opportunities for the repair and regeneration of lymphatic vessels [8].

This chapter offers a comprehensive review of the present landscape in bioengineering lymphatic vessels, concentrating on the design, creation, and utilization of bioengineered lymphatic structures. We start by examining the anatomy and physiology of the lymphatic system, then move on to an overview of the difficulties related to lymphatic vessel regeneration [9]. Next, we delve into the different methods employed in bioengineering lymphatic vessels, such as the application of biomaterials, cell-based therapies, and tissue engineering techniques [10]. Last, we discuss the possible clinical uses of bioengineered lymphatic vessels and the future prospects of this dynamic field [11].

2. Anatomy and physiology of the lymphatic system

The lymphatic system consists of a network of lymphatic vessels, lymph nodes, and lymphoid organs, such as the spleen, thymus, and tonsils [12]. Lymphatic vessels are delicate, valved structures that carry lymph—a fluid that includes white blood cells, proteins, and lipids—from the interstitial spaces of tissues back into the bloodstream [13]. This system is categorized into two primary parts: The superficial lymphatic system, which drains the skin and subcutaneous tissues, and the deep lymphatic system, which drains the muscles, joints, and internal organs [14].

2.1 Structure of lymphatic vessels

Lymphatic vessels consist of a single layer of endothelial cells, referred to as lymphatic endothelial cells (LECs), which are specialized for absorbing fluid and macromolecules from the interstitial space [15]. LECs are interconnected by tight junctions and are supported by a basement membrane along with adjacent pericytes [16]. Additionally, the lymphatic vessels contain valves that inhibit the backward flow of lymph, facilitating a one-way movement toward the lymph nodes and, ultimately, the venous system [17].

2.2 Functions of the lymphatic system

The lymphatic system is essential for immune monitoring, as it carries antigens and immune cells to the lymph nodes, where they can be processed and introduced to the immune response [18]. Moreover, the lymphatic system participates in the uptake of dietary fats from the digestive system and their delivery to the blood [19]. The lymphatic system also contributes to fluid balance by returning surplus interstitial fluid to the blood circulation, thus avoiding tissue swelling and edema [20].

3. Challenges in lymphatic vessel regeneration

Although the lymphatic system is crucial, the restoration of lymphatic vessels poses numerous difficulties. These difficulties arise from the intricate structure of the lymphatic network, the scarce presence of lymphatic endothelial cells (LECs), the fluid characteristics of the lymphatic system, and its close relationship with the immune system [21].

3.1 Intricacy of the lymphatic vessels

The lymphatic system consists of a structured network of vessels that vary in size, design, and purpose [22]. The restoration of lymphatic vessels necessitates an accurate reproduction of this intricate framework, which includes the development of operational valves and the association of the vessels with nearby tissues [3]. Reaching this degree of sophistication in bioengineered structures presents a considerable challenge [2].

3.2 Limited availability of LECs

LECs are challenging to isolate and grow *in vitro*, and their characteristics can quickly diminish during culture [15]. Furthermore, the process by which stem cells differentiate into LECs is not fully comprehended, and the elements that govern LEC differentiation and activity are still under investigation [16]. This restricted accessibility of LECs presents a major obstacle to advancing cell-based treatments for the regeneration of lymphatic vessels [17].

3.3 The fluidity of the lymphatic system

The lymphatic system is extremely active, with lymphatic vessels perpetually remodeling in response to changes in fluid homeostasis, inflammatory responses, and tissue restoration [18]. This ever-changing characteristic poses a difficulty for the development of bioengineered lymphatic structures, which need to adjust to the fluctuating microenvironment and connect with the host tissue [19].

3.4 Interaction with the immune system

The lymphatic system is intricately linked with the immune system; regeneration of lymphatic vessels can affect the functioning of the immune system [20]. The bioengineered lymphatic vessels should facilitate the movement of immune cells and the presentation of antigens, while simultaneously preventing the triggering of an immune reaction against the constructed tissue [21].

4. Approaches to bioengineering lymphatic vessels

4.1 Biomaterials for lymphatic vessel engineering

Biomaterials are essential in the creation and development of bioengineered lymphatic vessels. The perfect biomaterial for lymphatic vessel construction needs to be biocompatible, biodegradable, and capable of supporting the development and functionality of LECs [22]. Moreover, the biomaterial must possess mechanical characteristics that resemble those of natural lymphatic vessels, such as elasticity and compliance [3].

4.2 Natural polymers

Natural polymers, including collagen, fibrin, and hyaluronic acid, offer the benefits of biocompatibility and biodegradability, allowing them to create a natural extracellular matrix (ECM) setting for LECs [2]. Nonetheless, natural polymers can possess restricted mechanical strength and may experience swift degradation in vivo [15].

Feature	Natural polymers (e.g., collagen, fibrin, hyaluronic acid)	Synthetic polymers (e.g., PLGA, PCL, PEG)
Biocompatibility	Excellent; supports cell adhesion and growth	Good, but may require surface modification
Degradation rate	Rapid, often enzymatically degraded	Tunable, generally slower degradation
Mechanical strength	Lower; may need reinforcement	Higher; suitable for structural support
Immunogenicity	Potential immune response	Generally lower immune response
Fabrication control	Limited; batch variability	High control over structure and properties
Bioactivity	Inherent bioactive cues for cell signaling	Lacks bioactivity; may require functionalization
Applications in lymphatic engineering	Scaffolds, hydrogels for cell delivery	Tubular grafts, drug delivery systems

Table 1.
Comparison of natural and artificial polymers in lymphatic vessel engineering.

4.3 Synthetic polymers

Synthetic polymers, such as poly(lactic-co-glycolic acid) (PLGA), poly(ε-caprolactone) (PCL), and poly(glycerol sebacate) (PGS), provide enhanced regulation over mechanical attributes and degradation rates [16]. These substances can be constructed into scaffolds featuring specific designs, like microchannels or porous formations, that resemble the configuration of lymphatic vessels [17]. Nevertheless, synthetic polymers might be deficient in the biological signals required for LEC attachment, growth, and specialization [18].

4.4 Hybrid materials

Hybrid materials, which are a combination of natural and synthetic polymers, merge the benefits of both polymers [19]. For instance, a hybrid scaffold might consist of a synthetic polymer framework enveloped in a natural polymer to supply biological signals for LEC adherence and operation [20]. Furthermore, hybrid materials can be engineered to deliver growth factors or other bioactive compounds that facilitate the development and maturation of lymphatic vessels [21]. Here is an organized comparison chart of natural and synthetic polymers utilized in lymphatic vessel development (**Table 1**):

5. Cellular therapies for lymphatic vessel restoration

Cell-based treatments look promising for lymphatic vessel regeneration. The primary cell types utilized in lymphatic vessel development are LECs, which can be extracted from lymphatic tissues or developed from stem cells [22]. LECs may be placed onto biomaterial scaffolds or administered directly into the tissue to encourage the formation of new lymphatic vessels [3].

5.1 Stem cell differentiation

One of the obstacles to cell-based therapies is the restricted availability of LECs. To tackle this challenge, researchers have investigated the potential of stem cells, including mesenchymal stem cells (MSCs) and induced pluripotent stem cells (iPSCs), as a source of LECs [2]. Multiple studies have shown the ability of MSCs and iPSCs to transform into LECs through the application of various growth factors, such as vascular endothelial growth factor-C (VEGF-C) and fibroblast growth factor-2 (FGF-2) [15]. Nonetheless, the functional characteristics of the resulting LECs and the effectiveness of differentiation are still being improved and refined [16].

5.2 Progenitor cells

An alternative method for cell-based treatments involves utilizing progenitor cells, like lymphatic endothelial progenitor cells (LEPCs), that can evolve into lymphatic endothelial cells (LECs) and aid in forming lymphatic vessels [17]. LEPCs can be extracted from blood or bone marrow and subsequently expanded *in vitro* before their application in tissue engineering [18]. Nevertheless, the identification and extraction of LEPCs pose significant difficulties, and their function in the regeneration of lymphatic vessels is not yet fully comprehended [19].

6. Tissue engineering approaches for lymphatic vessel regeneration

Tissue engineering approaches for the regeneration of lymphatic vessels entail the creation of three-dimensional (3D) structures that replicate the design and function of natural lymphatic vessels [20]. These structures can be produced through various techniques, such as electrospinning, 3D printing, and microfluidics [21].

6.1 Electrospinning

Electrospinning is a method that employs an electric field to draw fibers from a polymer solution, leading to a fibrous framework with an extensive surface area and porosity [22]. Electrospun scaffolds can be created to replicate the structure of the lymphatic extracellular matrix and can be inserted with lymphatic endothelial cells to promote the formation of lymphatic vessels [3]. However, electrospun scaffolds might possess limited mechanical strength and might not entirely replicate the hierarchical architecture of lymphatic vessels [2].

6.2 3D printing

Three-dimensional printing, referred to as additive manufacturing, presents the capability to produce intricate 3D forms with accurate management of structure and materials [15]. This technology can be utilized to develop scaffolds featuring microchannels that replicate the architecture of lymphatic vessels, which can then be populated with LECs to encourage the development of vessels [16]. Moreover, 3D printing can also create layered structures that imitate the configuration of natural lymphatic vessels, encompassing the endothelial layer, basement membrane, and adjacent pericytes [17].

6.3 Microfluidics

Microfluidics is a method that utilizes micro-fabricated pathways to manage the movement of liquids on a microscale [18]. Microfluidic instruments can be employed to generate perfusable channels that replicate the architecture of lymphatic vessels, and these channels may be coated with LECs to develop operational lymphatic frameworks [19]. Microfluidic systems can additionally be utilized to study the behavior of LECs under regulated flow conditions, offering insights into the elements that govern lymphatic vessel development and operation [20].

7. Integration of bioengineered lymphatic vessels with host tissues

A major challenge in bioengineering lymphatic vessels is the incorporation of the engineered structures with the surrounding tissue. The bioengineered lymphatic vessels need to merge with the current lymphatic network and facilitate the movement of lymph [21]. Furthermore, the engineered vessels should have the capability to remodel and adjust to the evolving microenvironment, which includes variations in fluid balance, inflammation, and tissue healing [22].

7.1 Growth factors

Numerous methods have been employed to enhance the incorporation of bioengineered lymphatic vessels with surrounding tissues. One strategy involves utilizing growth factors, like VEGF-C and FGF-2, to encourage the development of new lymphatic vessels and the remodeling of current vessels [3]. These growth factors may be administered locally through biomaterial scaffolds or using controlled release systems [2].

7.2 Cell-based therapies

Another method involves utilizing cell-based treatments to enhance the incorporation of bioengineered lymphatic vessels. For instance, LECs or LEPCs can be administered into the area surrounding the engineered structure to encourage the development of new lymphatic vessels and the integration of the structure with the host tissue [15]. Furthermore, employing stem cells or progenitor cells could aid in tissue repair and remodeling, additionally improving the incorporation of the designed vessels [16].

7.3 Biomaterial scaffold design

Ultimately, the configuration of the biomaterial framework can be essential in facilitating the incorporation of bioengineered lymphatic vessels. Scaffolds featuring a porous or fibrous design can enhance cellular infiltration and tissue ingrowth, whereas scaffolds equipped with microchannels or perfusable networks can facilitate the development of functional lymphatic vessels [17]. Moreover, scaffolds that replicate the mechanical characteristics of natural lymphatic vessels may enhance the integration and remodeling of the designed vessels [18].

8. Clinical uses of bioengineered lymphatic vessels

8.1 Treatment of lymphedema

Lymphedema is a long-lasting condition defined by the buildup of lymphatic fluid within the tissues, resulting in swelling, fibrosis, and a compromised immune system [19]. Bioengineered lymphatic vessels present a hopeful solution for treating lymphedema. The insertion of bioengineered lymphatic structures may reinstate lymphatic circulation and alleviate swelling in the impacted tissues [20]. Moreover, bioengineered lymphatic vessels might serve to reconstruct damaged or missing lymphatic vessels after surgery or radiation treatment, preventing the onset of lymphedema [21].

8.2 Reconstruction of lymphatic vessels in cancer treatment

Cancer treatment, comprising surgical procedures, radiation treatment, and chemotherapy, may harm the lymphatic system, resulting in lymphedema and weakened immune response [22]. The repair of lymphatic vessels after cancer treatment can enhance patients' outcomes by reinstating lymphatic circulation and immune activity [3]. Furthermore, artificially created lymphatic vessels might be utilized to deliver therapeutic substances, including chemotherapy medications or immune modulators, straight to the tumor site, improving the effectiveness of cancer treatment [2].

8.3 Regeneration of lymphatic vessels in organ transplantation

Organ transplantation is a crucial procedure that saves the lives of individuals experiencing end-stage organ failure [15]. Nevertheless, the efficacy of organ transplantation can frequently be hindered by complications, including rejection and ischemia-reperfusion injury [16]. Enhancing the regeneration of lymphatic vessels in transplanted organs may lead to better graft survival by fostering immune tolerance and decreasing inflammation [17].

9. Future directions and conclusion

The domain of bioengineering lymphatic vessels remains in its foundational phases, yet it offers significant potential for addressing lymphatic conditions and progressing regenerative medicine [18]. Upcoming studies in this area should focus on various crucial aspects, such as the creation of innovative biomaterials, the enhancement of cell-centric therapies, and the incorporation of bioengineered lymphatic vessels with recipient tissues [19].

In summary, engineering lymphatic vessels signifies a novel realm in regenerative medicine, holding the promise to revolutionize the management of lymphatic disorders and enhance patient care [20]. Creating bioengineered lymphatic vessels will necessitate a collaborative strategy, merging knowledge from various fields like biomaterials, cell biology, tissue engineering, and clinical medicine [21]. With persistent research and advancements, bioengineered lymphatic vessels could evolve into a conventional therapy for various lymphatic ailments, providing hope for patients and propelling the progress of regenerative medicine [22].

Author details

Jyothsna Butchireddy
Omandurar Government College and Hospital, Chennai, India

*Address all correspondence to: jyothsnayadavredd@gmail.com

References

[1] Oliver G, Detmar M. The rediscovery of the lymphatic system: Old and new insights into the development and biological function of the lymphatic vasculature. Genes & Development. 2002;**16**(7):773-783

[2] Alitalo K. The lymphatic vasculature in disease. Nature Medicine. 2011;**17**(11):1371-1380

[3] Tammela T, Alitalo K. Lymphangiogenesis: Molecular mechanisms and future promise. Cell. 2010;**140**(4):460-476

[4] Randolph GJ, Ivanov S, Zinselmeyer BH, Scallan JP. The lymphatic system: Integral roles in immunity. Annual Review of Immunology. 2017;**35**:31-52

[5] Swartz MA. The physiology of the lymphatic system. Advanced Drug Delivery Reviews. 2001;**50**(1-2):3-20

[6] Rockson SG. Lymphedema. American Journal of Medicine. 2018;**131**(3):288-295

[7] Ji RC. Lymphatic endothelial cells, lymphangiogenesis, and extracellular matrix. Lymphatic Research and Biology. 2006;**4**(2):83-93

[8] Leak LV. The structure of lymphatic capillaries in lymph formation. Federation Proceedings. 1976;**35**(8):1863-1871

[9] Karpanen T, Alitalo K. Molecular biology and pathology of lymphangiogenesis. Annual Review of Pathology: Mechanisms of Disease. 2008;**3**:367-397

[10] Baluk P, Fuxe J, Hashizume H, et al. Functionally specialized junctions between endothelial cells of lymphatic vessels. Journal of Experimental Medicine. 2007;**204**(10):2349-2362

[11] Petrova TV, Koh GY. Biological functions of lymphatic vessels. Science. 2020;**369**(6500):eaax4063

[12] Aspelund A, Robciuc MR, Karaman S, et al. Lymphatic system in cardiovascular medicine. Circulation Research. 2016;**118**(3):515-530

[13] Alitalo K, Tammela T, Petrova TV. Lymphangiogenesis in development and human disease. Nature. 2005;**438**(7070):946-953

[14] Schulte-Merker S, Sabine A, Petrova TV. Lymphatic vascular morphogenesis in development, physiology, and disease. Journal of Cell Biology. 2011;**193**(4):607-618

[15] Oliver G, Srinivasan RS. Endothelial cell plasticity: How to become and remain a lymphatic endothelial cell. Development. 2010;**137**(3):363-372

[16] Wigle JT, Oliver G. Prox1 function is required for the development of the murine lymphatic system. Cell. 1999;**98**(6):769-778

[17] Jurisic G, Detmar M. Lymphatic endothelium in health and disease. Cell and Tissue Research. 2009;**335**(1):97-108

[18] Randolph GJ, Angeli V, Swartz MA. Dendritic-cell trafficking to lymph nodes through lymphatic vessels. Nature Reviews Immunology. 2005;**5**(8):617-628

[19] Bernier-Latmani J, Petrova TV. Intestinal lymphatic vasculature: Structure, mechanisms and functions.

Nature Reviews Gastroenterology & Hepatology. 2017;**14**(9):510-526

[20] Rockson SG. Lymphedema. American Journal of Medicine. 2001;**110**(4):288-295

[21] Cueni LN, Detmar M. The lymphatic system in health and disease. Lymphatic Research and Biology. 2008;**6**(3-4):109-122

[22] Karaman S, Detmar M. Mechanisms of lymphatic metastasis. Journal of Clinical Investigation. 2014;**124**(3):922-928

Chapter 5

Advances in the Pathophysiology, Diagnosis, and Treatment of Lymphomas: A Comprehensive Overview

Maaweya Jabareen, Muhammad Al-Sweity, Wasef Alhroub, Kenana Altel and Abdalqader Aljaradat

Abstract

This comprehensive overview delves into the pathophysiology, diagnosis, and treatment of lymphomas, focusing on Hodgkin and non-Hodgkin subtypes. The text explores genetic alterations, environmental triggers, and immune dysregulation that drive lymphomagenesis. Hodgkin lymphoma (HL) features Reed-Sternberg cells, with subtypes requiring tailored chemoradiotherapy or immunotherapy. Non-Hodgkin lymphoma (NHL) spans diverse B-cell, T-cell, and NK-cell malignancies, including aggressive forms like diffuse large B-cell lymphoma (DLBCL) and indolent variants such as follicular lymphoma. Advances in targeted therapies, including monoclonal antibodies, CAR-T cell therapy, and stem cell transplantation, have transformed treatment paradigms, enhancing outcomes for refractory cases. Emerging biomarkers and genetic profiling enable precision medicine approaches, addressing the unique molecular and clinical landscapes of various subtypes. Despite progress, challenges persist in managing relapsed or high-risk lymphomas, underscoring the need for ongoing research into innovative treatments.

Keywords: lymphoma, Hodgkin lymphoma, non-Hodgkin lymphoma, pathophysiology, diagnosis, targeted therapy, CAR-T cell therapy, immunotherapy

1. Introduction

Lymphomas are a diverse group of cancers that originate from the clonal expansion of B cells, T cells, or natural killer (NK) cells, affecting lymphocytes at various stages of their maturation [1]. Lymphomas can be broadly classified into two main categories: non-Hodgkin lymphoma (NHL), which accounts for approximately 90% of cases, and Hodgkin lymphoma (HL), representing the remaining 10%. The majority of lymphomas, around 90%, arise from B cells [2]. Lymphoid neoplasms rank as the fourth most prevalent type of cancer and are the sixth leading cause of cancer-related deaths in the United States [3].

The pathophysiology of lymphoma involves genetic alterations in lymphocytes, which disrupt the normal regulation of their growth and division, leading to uncontrolled proliferation. Various stressors, including infections, chronic inflammation, and exposure to toxic agents, further drive this abnormal process. A critical aspect of lymphoma development is prolonged immunosuppression, which compromises the innate immune system's ability to detect and eliminate malignant cells or respond to infections that may trigger cancer formation [1, 4].

2. Classification

Hodgkin lymphoma (HL) is diagnosed in approximately 8540 cases annually in the U.S., with bimodal age peaks. While its exact cause is unclear, associated factors include familial predisposition, Epstein-Barr virus (EBV) infections, and immune suppression [5]. HL has two main subtypes: *classical HL (cHL)*, accounting for 90% of cases, and *nodular lymphocyte-predominant HL (NLPHL)*. cHL features Reed-Sternberg cells, CD15/CD30 positivity, and four histologic subtypes, while NLPHL involves CD20-positive lymphocyte-predominant cells, Epstein-Barr Virus (EBV) is typically absent, and NLPHL lacks classic Reed-Sternberg cells [6].

Risk factors for HL include EBV, HIV, genetic predisposition, and socioeconomic status, with higher incidence in developed regions [7]. The disease commonly presents as painless lymphadenopathy, often in the neck or mediastinum, with advanced cases showing B symptoms like fever and weight loss [6]. *Staging* uses PET-CT and divides HL into limited (stages I-II) or advanced (stages III-IV) categories [8]. *Pathophysiology* involves malignant Reed-Sternberg cells originating from B cells with disrupted signaling pathways like JAK/STAT and NF-κB, with EBV playing a role in some cases. HL is histologically marked by Reed-Sternberg cells and distinct features across subtypes, such as sclerosis in nodular sclerosis cHL, with immune evasion mechanisms supporting tumor survival [9].

Treatment of cHL includes chemotherapy (ABVD or BEACOPP) and radiation, with risk-adapted approaches guided by interim PET scans. Relapsed cases are treated with salvage chemotherapy, autologous stem-cell transplantation, or immunotherapy [6]. NLPHL treatment varies by stage, with radiation for early disease and chemotherapy (e.g., R-CHOP) for advanced or relapsed cases [10]. *Prognosis* is excellent for early-stage disease, with cure rates of 90–95%, though advanced cases have lower survival [7]. *Complications* include secondary malignancies, cardiopulmonary toxicity, and infertility, requiring long-term follow-up [6]. NLPHL patients, while having indolent disease, may face late relapses or transformation to aggressive lymphomas like DLBCL [11].

In contrast, NHL comprises a wide range of subtypes which include mature *B cells, T and NK neoplasms* with diffuse large B-cell lymphoma (DLBCL) which is a subtype of NHL being the most common and aggressive form, making up about 30% of NHL cases [12]. Mature B-cell lymphomas are a heterogeneous group of disorders with diverse clinical presentations, genetic abnormalities, and outcomes. These malignancies arise from various stages of B-cell differentiation and involve distinct therapeutic approaches and include the following:

Chronic lymphocytic leukemia (CLL) and small lymphocytic lymphoma (SLL) are the same disease involving mature B lymphocytes, with CLL being the most common adult leukemia in Western countries, primarily affecting individuals over 70. Diagnosis involves blood tests, bone marrow analysis, and immunophenotyping, with management ranging from active surveillance to targeted therapies, chemotherapy, or stem cell transplantation for progressive cases [13].

Monoclonal B-cell lymphocytosis (MBL) is a premalignant condition with clonal B cells resembling CLL but without disease symptoms. It has low-count and high-count subtypes, with high-count MBL carrying a 1-2% annual progression risk to CLL. Key factors include cytogenetic abnormalities like del(13q14), advanced age, male gender, and genetic predisposition. High-count MBL requires annual monitoring, while low-count MBL usually remains stable [14].

B-cell prolymphocytic leukemia (B-PLL) is a rare, aggressive B-cell malignancy affecting older adults, characterized by a high proportion of prolymphocytes, MYC and TP53 mutations, and aggressive B-cell proliferation. Prolymphocytes have prominent nucleoli and basophilic cytoplasm. Diagnosis relies on leukocytosis and splenomegaly. Treatment includes targeted therapies, combination regimens, and stem cell transplantation, but prognosis is poor, with a median survival of about 3 years [15].

Splenic marginal zone lymphoma (SMZL) is an indolent lymphoma involving the spleen and bone marrow, linked to chronic antigenic stimulation like hepatitis C virus (HCV) infection, with antigen-driven B-cell proliferation and del(7q) and NOTCH2 mutations. Treatment includes watchful waiting, rituximab monotherapy, or splenectomy, with a median survival of 10–15 years, but prognosis worsens with transformation to aggressive lymphoma [16].

Hairy cell leukemia (HCL) is a rare B-cell malignancy with pancytopenia, splenomegaly, and hairy cells in blood smears. It involves the BRAF V600E mutation, activating the MAPK/ERK pathway. Histopathology shows "fried egg" cells in bone marrow with CD20, CD103, and CD25 markers. Treatment with purine analogs leads to high remission rates, but relapses may need BRAF inhibitors. Prognosis is excellent for classic HCL, but the variant form is more aggressive [17, 18].

Splenic B-cell lymphoma/leukemia, unclassifiable, includes rare low-grade B-cell disorders like splenic diffuse red pulp lymphoma and hairy cell leukemia variant. It involves clonal B-cell proliferation with mutations such as IGLL5 and KMT2D. Histopathology shows diffuse infiltration of the splenic red pulp by small B cells. Symptoms include splenomegaly and cytopenias. Treatment options are splenectomy, rituximab, and chemotherapy, with prognosis depending on disease progression and complications [19].

Splenic diffuse red pulp small B-cell lymphoma (SDRPL) is a rare indolent lymphoma with diffuse splenic red pulp infiltration, and it involves B-cell proliferation driven by mutations like NOTCH1 and TP53. Symptoms include splenomegaly, lymphocytosis, and cytopenias, with treatment options such as splenectomy, rituximab, and chemoimmunotherapy, and a generally favorable prognosis that worsens with progression [20, 21].

Hairy cell leukemia-variant (HCL-v) is an aggressive disorder lacking the BRAF V600E mutation, with dysregulated MAPK/BCR signaling and TP53 abnormalities. It presents with splenomegaly, elevated leukocytes, and chemoresistance. Treatment includes purine analogs with rituximab, and research is exploring MEK inhibitors. Prognosis is poorer than classic HCL, with frequent relapses [22].

Lymphoplasmacytic lymphoma (Waldenström macroglobulinemia) is an indolent lymphoma with IgM monoclonal gammopathy and bone marrow infiltration. Pathophysiology involves MYD88 L265P and CXCR4 mutations. Histopathology shows infiltration by lymphoplasmacytic cells expressing CD19, CD20, and IgM. Symptoms include hyperviscosity, fatigue, and anemia. Treatment includes BTK inhibitors, chemoimmunotherapy, and plasmapheresis. Prognosis depends on mutation status and risk stratification [23, 24].

Monoclonal gammopathy of undetermined significance (MGUS), IgM: It is a premalignant condition with low progression risk to Waldenström macroglobulinemia or other lymphoproliferative disorders. Pathophysiology involves clonal B-cell expansion with MYD88 mutations. Bone marrow shows less than 10% lymphoplasmacytic infiltration. Most cases remain stable, but monitoring is essential. Symptoms, like hyperviscosity or neuropathy, are treated with targeted therapies [25, 26].

Heavy-chain diseases (μ-HCD and γ-HCD) are rare disorders with truncated immunoglobulin heavy chains and no light chains. Pathophysiology involves mutations in the immunoglobulin gene, causing abnormal heavy-chain production and clonal B-cell proliferation. μ-HCD resembles CLL and is linked to MYD88 mutations, while γ-HCD is associated with autoimmune diseases and EBV infections. Histopathology shows plasma cells with aberrant heavy-chain expression. Treatment includes rituximab-based regimens for μ-HCD or CHOP for γ-HCD. Prognosis worsens with advanced disease or lymphoma transformation [27, 28].

High-grade B-cell lymphomas with MYC and BCL2/BCL6 rearrangements ("double-hit" or "triple-hit") are aggressive malignancies with poor outcomes. Pathophysiology involves genetic rearrangements disrupting apoptosis and cell proliferation. Histopathology resembles DLBCL with high MYC and BCL2 expression. Treatment includes intensified chemotherapy and CNS prophylaxis, with novel therapies being explored. HGBL-NOS, another subtype, lacks MYC rearrangements but requires similar management [29, 30].

Gray-zone lymphoma (GZL) is a rare lymphoma with features of both DLBCL and classical Hodgkin lymphoma. Pathophysiology involves MYC and BCL2 rearrangements. Histopathology shows Reed-Sternberg-like cells expressing CD30 and B-cell markers. It often presents as a mediastinal mass in young adults. Treatment includes chemotherapy and radiotherapy, but prognosis is poor due to frequent relapses and aggressive progression [31, 32].

EBV+ mucocutaneous ulcer is a rare, indolent B-cell neoplasm linked to immunosenescence or immunosuppression, primarily affecting older individuals, HIV patients, and transplant recipients, presenting as mucosal or cutaneous ulcers. The prognosis is favorable with a low risk of systemic progression, and most cases regress after reducing immunosuppression, though severe cases may require radiotherapy or rituximab [33, 34].

Diffuse large B-cell lymphoma (DLBCL) is the most common type, often arising from chronic inflammation like rheumatoid arthritis, hepatitis C, or inflammatory bowel disease. It presents with swollen lymph nodes, fever, weight loss, and fatigue. Histopathology shows large, atypical lymphocytes. Treatment is R-CHOP chemotherapy, with radiation for localized disease. Prognosis depends on treatment response, but inflammation can complicate management, with long-term risks of relapse and therapy resistance [35, 36].

Lymphomatoid granulomatosis is a rare angiocentric lymphoproliferative disorder linked to EBV and immune dysfunction, affecting adults and immunodeficient children. Symptoms include cough, dyspnea, fever, and neurological issues. Treatment includes interferon-alpha for low-grade disease and DA-EPOCH-R chemotherapy for high-grade cases. Relapse and progression to aggressive lymphoma are common [35].

Primary mediastinal large B-cell lymphoma (PMBL) is an aggressive lymphoma originating in the thymus, typically affecting young adults, and presents with symptoms like cough, dyspnea, and superior vena cava syndrome due to bulky mediastinal masses. Treatment includes R-EPOCH chemotherapy, with autologous stem cell transplant or CAR-T for refractory cases, and prognosis is favorable if detected early, though complications may arise [37].

Intravascular large B-cell lymphoma is a rare and aggressive subtype characterized by the proliferation of lymphoma cells within blood vessels. Symptoms include fever, weight loss, and organ dysfunction (e.g., CNS, lungs). Treatment includes rituximab-based chemotherapy, but prognosis remains poor due to frequent delayed diagnoses and complications like organ failure and hemophagocytic syndrome [38].

Anaplastic lymphoma kinase-positive large B-cell lymphoma is a rare, aggressive form defined by ALK gene translocation and STAT3 pathway activation, affecting young, immunocompetent men with widespread lymphadenopathy. Histopathology shows immunoblast-like cells with plasmablastic differentiation, and treatment typically involves CHOP or E-POCH chemotherapy. Prognosis is generally poor, though localized disease in children shows better outcomes, with complications including bone marrow involvement, relapse, and secondary infections [39].

Plasmablastic lymphoma is an aggressive B-cell lymphoma associated with immunodeficiency, particularly in HIV patients. It predominantly affects extranodal sites like the oral cavity. Pathophysiology involves post-germinal center plasmablasts. Histopathology reveals monomorphic plasmablastic cells. Treatment includes V-EPOCH chemotherapy, but prognosis is poor, with frequent relapses and short survival. Complications include disease spread, infections, and chemotherapy-related toxicity [40].

Primary effusion lymphoma (PEL) is a rare lymphoma linked to HHV8 and EBV infections, affecting serous cavities without lymphadenopathy, often presenting in HIV patients. Treatment includes chemotherapy (e.g., DA-EPOCH) with antiretroviral therapy, but prognosis is poor, with median survival under 2 years and complications like systemic spread and severe immunosuppression [41].

HHV8+ diffuse large B-cell lymphoma (DLBCL) is an aggressive neoplasm involving HHV8-infected plasmablastic cells, primarily occurring in immunocompromised individuals like HIV-positive patients, often associated with multicentric Castleman disease. Treatment follows regimens for HIV-associated DLBCL, but prognosis is poor due to the aggressive nature of the disease and frequent relapses [42].

Burkitt lymphoma is a highly aggressive B-cell lymphoma characterized by c-MYC gene translocation, presenting in endemic, sporadic, and immunodeficiency-related subtypes. Treatment includes intensive chemotherapy with CNS prophylaxis, and prognosis is excellent in high-income settings but remains poor in low-resource areas [43].

Alpha heavy-chain disease (α-HCD), or immunoproliferative small intestinal disease, is a rare B-cell neoplasm producing defective monoclonal heavy chains. It is linked to chronic intestinal infections like *Campylobacter jejuni*. Symptoms include malabsorption, diarrhea, and weight loss. Histopathology shows plasma cell infiltration in the bowel mucosa. Early stages respond to antibiotics, while advanced cases require chemotherapy. Prognosis depends on disease stage, with risks of severe malnutrition and progression to diffuse large B-cell lymphoma [44, 45].

Monoclonal gammopathy of undetermined significance (MGUS) is a premalignant condition characterized by monoclonal protein production without organ damage, commonly occurring in older adults and African Americans. Diagnosis is incidental and confirmed by serum protein analysis, with management involving regular monitoring and treatment initiated upon progression, as the annual progression risk is ~1%, requiring long-term follow-up [46, 47].

Plasma cell myeloma (multiple myeloma) is a malignant disorder of plasma cells producing excessive monoclonal proteins, leading to bone destruction, renal impairment, and anemia, with symptoms including bone pain, fractures, recurrent infections, and hypercalcemia. Treatment includes chemotherapy, immunotherapy, and stem cell transplantation, but complications such as bone damage and organ dysfunction pose significant challenges [48, 49].

Solitary plasmacytoma of bone is a localized plasma cell tumor without systemic involvement, commonly affecting men aged ~68 and presenting with bone pain or mass-related symptoms. Treatment typically involves localized radiation therapy, and up to two-thirds of cases progress to multiple myeloma, requiring close monitoring for systemic spread [50, 51].

Extraosseous plasmacytoma is a plasma cell tumor occurring in soft tissues, often in the upper respiratory or gastrointestinal tract, with symptoms varying based on location. Treatment includes radiation therapy, and the disease generally has a good prognosis, though a small percentage progress to multiple myeloma [51, 52].

MALT lymphoma is an indolent B-cell lymphoma associated with chronic inflammation, often due to *Helicobacter pylori* infection, primarily affecting the stomach. Treatment involves eradicating *H. pylori*, with chemotherapy or radiation for refractory cases, and prognosis is favorable, though some cases transform into diffuse large B-cell lymphoma [53, 54].

Pediatric nodal marginal zone lymphoma is a rare pediatric lymphoma with expanded marginal zones, and it typically presents as localized nodal enlargement in the head and neck. Histopathology shows polymorphous cellular infiltrates with monocytoid and plasmacytoid cells. The disease is indolent, with excellent survival rates (~100%) after surgical excision or conservative treatment. Relapses are rare, and systemic involvement is uncommon [55, 56].

In situ follicular neoplasia is a premalignant condition marked by BCL2-positive B cells confined to germinal centers. It is often detected incidentally and has a low risk of progression to follicular lymphoma. Histopathology shows intact lymph node architecture with BCL2 and CD10 positivity. No treatment is required for isolated findings, but monitoring is essential for detecting progression [57].

Duodenal-type follicular lymphoma is an indolent lymphoma occurring in the duodenum, often detected incidentally during endoscopy, with histopathology showing lymphoid aggregates sparing the muscularis propria. Treatment ranges from watchful waiting to localized radiation, with an excellent prognosis and a low risk of progression to nodal disease or systemic involvement [58].

Pediatric-type follicular lymphoma is a rare lymphoma affecting children and young adults, presenting with localized lymphadenopathy, often in the head and neck. Histopathology shows blastoid cells in expanded follicles, with treatment involving surgical excision and, in rare cases, chemotherapy or radiation, offering an excellent prognosis and minimal risk of progression or relapse [59].

Large B-cell lymphoma with IRF4 rearrangement is a rare lymphoma primarily affecting children and young adults, often involving the Waldeyer ring. It shows IRF4 gene rearrangement and MUM1 expression. Histopathology reveals diffuse or follicular patterns with medium to large lymphoid cells. Treatment involves immunochemotherapy, yielding favorable outcomes. Relapse and treatment-related complications remain concerns [60, 61].

Primary cutaneous follicle center lymphoma is a low-grade lymphoma arising in the skin, and it presents as nodules or plaques, often on the scalp or trunk. Histopathology reveals centrocytes and centroblasts in the dermis. Localized radiation or surgery achieves excellent outcomes, with rare extracutaneous spread. Recurrence is observed in ~30% of cases [62].

In situ mantle cell neoplasia: A premalignant condition involving cyclin D1-positive B cells confined to mantle zones. It is often detected incidentally. Progression to mantle cell lymphoma is rare (<10%). Histopathology shows preserved lymphoid architecture with minimal mantle zone expansion. Management involves monitoring, with treatment initiated only if progression occurs [63, 64].

Diffuse large B-cell lymphoma, NOS, is an aggressive lymphoma with subtypes (GCB and ABC). It presents as rapidly enlarging masses with or without B symptoms. Pathophysiology involves de novo occurrence or transformation from low-grade lymphomas. Treatment includes R-CHOP chemotherapy. Complications include relapse, infections, and organ involvement [65].

Primary cutaneous CD30-positive T-cell lymphoproliferative disorders include *lymphomatoid papulosis (LyP)* and *primary cutaneous anaplastic large cell lymphoma (PC-ALCL)*. *LyP* is a chronic, self-healing condition characterized by recurrent erythematous papules and nodules, often on the trunk and extremities, with spontaneous regression and low treatment needs. Treatment includes PUVA, corticosteroids, brentuximab vedotin, and low-dose methotrexate, with an excellent prognosis, but there is a risk of secondary lymphoid malignancies and chronic relapses [66]. *PC-ALCL* presents as localized or multifocal nodules, sometimes ulcerated, with CD30+ anaplastic malignant cells and cohesive dermal tumor infiltrates. Treatment includes radiotherapy or excision for localized lesions, and methotrexate or brentuximab vedotin for multifocal disease, with a favorable prognosis and a 90% 10-year survival rate, though 10% may experience extracutaneous spread [67].

Primary cutaneous gamma-delta T-cell lymphoma (PCGD-TCL) is a rare and aggressive lymphoma caused by clonal proliferation of mature gamma-delta T cells, presenting as rapidly progressing plaques or ulceronecrotic nodules. It is resistant to chemotherapy, and allogeneic hematopoietic stem cell transplantation offers the only potential benefit, with a poor prognosis and a median survival of 15 months [68].

Primary cutaneous CD8+ aggressive epidermotropic cytotoxic T-cell lymphoma (PCAECTCL) is a rare, aggressive subtype of cutaneous T-cell lymphoma with significant epidermotropism of cytotoxic T cells, leading to epidermal necrosis and ulceration. It presents as rapidly progressing ulcerative nodules or plaques, with limited responses to chemotherapy and stem cell transplantation, and a median survival of less than 2 years [46].

Burkitt-like lymphoma with 11q aberration (BLL-11q) mimics Burkitt lymphoma but lacks MYC rearrangements, showing 11q aberration with proximal gains and telomeric losses. It primarily affects children and young adults, presenting as a bulky tumor with localized lymphadenopathy, and is treated with intensive chemoimmunotherapy with CNS prophylaxis. Prognosis is favorable, with an 80% 5-year survival rate, similar to Burkitt lymphoma [69].

Mature T and NK neoplasms

T-cell prolymphocytic leukemia (T-PLL) is a rare, aggressive malignancy of mature T-lymphocytes, primarily affecting older adults (median age 65), with a slight male predominance. It is driven by genetic mutations, including TCL1 overexpression and frequent ATM mutations, leading to genomic instability. Despite treatments like alemtuzumab and stem cell transplantation, prognosis is poor, with a median survival of about 19 months [70].

T-cell large granular lymphocytic leukemia (T-LGLL) is a rare, indolent lymphoproliferative disorder affecting individuals aged 66 and older, driven by JAK/STAT activation and STAT3 mutations in 40%-50% of cases. Clinical features include neutropenia, anemia, and splenomegaly, with immunosuppressive therapies managing symptoms and a 10-year survival rate of about 64% [71].

Chronic lymphoproliferative disorder of NK cells (CLPD-NK) is a rare hematologic disorder affecting adults over 60, with a slight female predominance, often discovered during evaluations for persistent lymphocytosis. Symptomatic cases may cause cytopenias, splenomegaly, recurrent infections, and skin lesions, with viral infections and STAT3 mutations leading to clonal NK cell expansion, and management involves monitoring asymptomatic cases and immunosuppressive therapies, with a 5-year survival rate of ~94% [72].

Aggressive NK-cell leukemia (ANKL) is a rare and fatal malignancy linked to EBV and STAT3 mutations, primarily affecting Asian males around 42 years old, presenting with fever, hepatosplenomegaly, and cytopenias. Marked by medium-to-large lymphoid cells and EBV positivity, treatments like SMILE and HSCT offer limited benefit, with a median survival of less than 2 months [73].

Systemic EBV+ T-cell lymphoma of childhood is a rare, aggressive malignancy arising from EBV-infected cytotoxic T cells, primarily affecting Asian populations. It presents with fever, hepatosplenomegaly, lymphadenopathy, and multiorgan failure, with treatment including CHOP-like or SMILE chemotherapy and allogeneic HSCT, but prognosis remains poor due to rapid progression and fatal outcomes [74].

Hydroa vacciniforme-like lymphoproliferative disorder (HV-LPD) is a rare lymphoproliferative disorder linked to chronic Epstein-Barr virus (EBV) infection, and it primarily affects children and adolescents in Asia and Latin America. It presents with papulovesicular skin lesions, fever, and lymphadenopathy, with treatment including antiviral, steroid, and stem cell transplantation, and prognosis varying from indolent to aggressive systemic lymphoma, especially in adults [75].

Adult T-cell leukemia/lymphoma (ATLL) is a rare malignancy caused by chronic human T-lymphotropic virus type 1 (HTLV-1) infection, primarily in endemic areas like Japan and the Caribbean. It has four subtypes: acute, lymphomatous, chronic, and smoldering, with acute and lymphomatous forms being aggressive and presenting with systemic symptoms. Management includes chemotherapy, antiviral therapy, and stem cell transplantation, with prognosis varying from poor for aggressive forms (9–13 months) to better for indolent types (2–4 years) [76, 77].

Extranodal NK/T-cell lymphoma, nasal type (ENKTCL-NT), is an aggressive cancer linked to Epstein-Barr virus (EBV), more common in East Asia and among Native Americans, with a male predominance, presenting with nasal obstruction, nosebleeds, and facial swelling. Treatment includes radiation for localized disease and chemotherapy regimens like SMILE for advanced stages, with prognosis varying based on stage [78].

Enteropathy-associated T-cell lymphoma (EATL) is a rare, aggressive cancer linked to celiac disease and HLA-DQ2 homozygosity, arising from intraepithelial lymphocytes in the small intestine due to chronic inflammation and JAK/STAT pathway mutations. Treatment involves surgery, chemotherapy, and autologous stem cell transplantation, but prognosis is poor with a median survival of 6 to 10 months [79].

Monomorphic epitheliotropic intestinal T-cell lymphoma (MEITL) is a rare and aggressive form of primary intestinal T-cell lymphoma arises from intraepithelial lymphocytes in the gastrointestinal tract, not associated with celiac disease. It presents with abdominal pain, weight loss, and gastrointestinal bleeding and has a poor prognosis with a median survival of less than 6 months [80].

Indolent T-cell lymphoproliferative disorder of the gastrointestinal tract (iTLPD-GI) is a rare condition characterized by the clonal proliferation of mature T-cells in the gastrointestinal tract, affecting the small intestine and colon, with symptoms like abdominal pain, diarrhea, and weight loss. Involving mutations in genes like STAT3-JAK2, it requires treatment including radiotherapy, and while the prognosis is generally favorable, some cases may progress to more aggressive lymphomas [81].

Hepatosplenic T-cell lymphoma (HSTCL) is a rare, aggressive peripheral T-cell lymphoma affects young adult males and is often linked to long-term immunosuppression. It is characterized by $\gamma\delta$ T-cell infiltration into the liver, spleen, and bone marrow, with poor prognosis and a median survival of 11 months, though aggressive treatment like HyperCVAD chemotherapy and hematopoietic stem cell transplantation can improve survival [82, 83].

Subcutaneous panniculitis-like T-cell lymphoma (SPTCL) is a rare non-Hodgkin lymphoma, more common in Asian populations, linked to autoimmune conditions, and involves cytotoxic T-cells causing panniculitis and subcutaneous nodules. Treatment includes corticosteroids, chemotherapy, and stem cell transplants, with a generally favorable prognosis, though hemophagocytic syndrome can worsen outcomes [84, 85].

Mycosis fungoides (MF) and Sézary syndrome (SS) are primary cutaneous T-cell lymphomas, comprise 70-85% of primary cutaneous lymphomas, with MF causing persistent pruritic skin lesions and SS presenting with diffuse lesions, lymphadenopathy, and systemic symptoms. Treatments include topical corticosteroids, chemotherapy, and stem cell transplants, with early-stage MF having a favorable prognosis, while SS has a poor prognosis and a 5-year survival rate around 42% [86, 87].

Primary cutaneous CD4+ small/medium T-cell lymphoproliferative disorder (PCSM-TCLPD) is a subtype of primary cutaneous T-cell lymphoma (CTCL), accounting for 8–12% of cases, and is characterized by CD4+ pleomorphic T cells without mycosis fungoides-like lesions. Patients typically present with solitary plaques or tumors, treated with intralesional steroids, surgical excision, or radiotherapy, with an excellent prognosis and rare recurrences [46, 88].

Peripheral T-cell lymphoma, not otherwise specified (PTCL-NOS), is a heterogeneous lymphoma accounting for 30% of PTCL cases and 4% of NHLs, with an increasing incidence in Western countries. It typically presents with lymphadenopathy and extranodal involvement, including skin and gastrointestinal tract, and is treated with CHOEP chemotherapy and autologous stem-cell transplantation, with a poor prognosis and 5-year OS of 28-35% [89].

Angioimmunoblastic T-cell lymphoma (AITL) is a distinct PTCL subtype representing 15–20% of cases. It affects older adults and presents with systemic symptoms, lymphadenopathy, and rash. Histopathology shows diffuse infiltrates with prominent endothelial venules and regressed follicles. Treatment includes CHOP chemotherapy and autologous stem-cell transplantation. The 5-year survival rate is 32%, reflecting poor prognosis [90, 91].

Follicular peripheral T-cell lymphoma (F-PTCL) is a rare PTCL subtype, affecting older males. It presents with B-symptoms and advanced nodal disease. Histopathology shows follicular growth patterns with neoplastic cells in lymphoid follicles. Biomarker-targeted therapies, including CAR-T-cell therapy, are emerging. Prognosis is poor due to the presence of T-follicular helper cells [92].

Nodal peripheral T-cell lymphoma with T follicular helper (TFH) phenotype is an aggressive lymphoma primarily involves lymph nodes and is defined by TFH markers and RHOA mutations. Patients present with advanced disease and lymphadenopathy. Histopathology shows tumor cell-rich infiltration in lymph nodes. Treatment includes CHOP chemotherapy and epigenetic modifiers. Prognosis is better than PTCL-NOS but still poor [93, 94].

Anaplastic large cell lymphoma (ALCL), ALK Positive, is a CD30-positive T-cell lymphoma common in young individuals. It is characterized by hallmark cells with horseshoe nuclei. The ALK gene drives oncogenesis. Patients often present with advanced disease and B symptoms. Treatment includes CHOP chemotherapy and ALK inhibitors. ALK-positive cases have a 5-year survival rate of 80% [95].

Anaplastic large cell lymphoma, ALK negative, is a lymphoma that is similar to ALK-positive ALCL but lacks ALK expression. It affects older adults and presents with advanced-stage disease. Treatment includes CHOP chemotherapy and brentuximab vedotin. Prognosis is worse than ALK-positive cases [96].

Breast implant-associated anaplastic large cell lymphoma (BIA-ALCL) is a lymphoma that arises around textured breast implants. It is linked to chronic antigen stimulation. Patients present with effusion, rash, or masses. Localized disease is treated with capsulectomy, while invasive cases may require chemotherapy. Prognosis varies based on disease extent [97].

3. Summary

The prognosis and outcomes of lymphoma vary widely based on subtype, disease stage at diagnosis, patient age, and overall health. Hodgkin's lymphoma generally has a favorable prognosis, with over 80% of patients achieving five-year survival with current treatments, which include chemotherapy and radiation [6]. NHL prognosis, however, differs based on subtype and stage. Aggressive lymphomas like DLBCL have a five-year survival rate of about 60%, while indolent lymphomas like follicular lymphoma may have a prolonged survival but are often considered incurable [98]. Prognostic markers, such as advanced age, high lactate dehydrogenase (LDH) levels, the presence of B symptoms, and certain genetic mutations, significantly affect survival. For example, the presence of MYC gene rearrangements in Burkitt lymphoma is associated with poorer outcomes [6, 98].

Lymphoma treatment is carefully tailored to the subtype and stage of disease. Chemotherapy remains the mainstay treatment, with the ABVD regimen (adriamycin, bleomycin, vinblastine, and dacarbazine) being standard for Hodgkin's lymphoma [99, 100]. For aggressive NHL forms like DLBCL, the R-CHOP regimen (rituximab, cyclophosphamide, hydroxydaunorubicin, oncovin, and prednisone) is commonly used [101]. Radiation therapy often complements chemotherapy, especially in early-stage HL and localized NHL cases. Targeted therapies, such as monoclonal antibodies like Rituximab, have greatly improved outcomes in B-cell lymphomas. Immunotherapy, including checkpoint inhibitors and CAR-T cell therapy, has shown promise in treating relapsed or refractory lymphomas. CAR-T cell therapy, which modifies a patient's T-cells to specifically target lymphoma cells, has been particularly effective for aggressive lymphomas like DLBCL and mantle cell lymphoma that do not respond to conventional treatments [100, 102].

Stem cell transplantation represents another vital treatment option, especially for relapsed or refractory lymphoma cases. Autologous stem cell transplantation, where the patient's own stem cells are used, is frequently employed for relapsed Hodgkin's lymphoma and aggressive NHL. In high-risk cases, allogeneic stem cell transplantation (using donor stem cells) may be considered, though it carries a higher risk of complications such as graft-versus-host disease [103, 104].

Despite progress, patients with relapsed or refractory lymphoma still face challenges. New therapies, including small molecule inhibitors like Bruton's tyrosine kinase (BTK) inhibitors and bispecific antibodies that engage both T cells and lymphoma cells, are currently being studied in clinical trials and offer hope for improving outcomes in these difficult cases [105]. As research further illuminates the molecular mechanisms underlying lymphoma, personalized treatment approaches based on the tumor's genetic and immunologic profile are likely to become increasingly central in managing this diverse group of cancers.

4. Conclusions

Lymphoma is a complex, heterogeneous disease encompassing a wide range of subtypes, each with distinct risk factors, clinical features, and treatment outcomes. While substantial progress has been made in understanding and treating lymphoma, ongoing research into novel therapies and personalized approaches remains essential to further improve patient outcomes. Identifying genetic and environmental risk factors, refining treatment strategies, and developing innovative therapies will be critical in reducing the global impact of lymphoma.

Acknowledgements

The author acknowledges the use of ChatGPT for language polishing of the manuscript.

Author details

Maaweya Jabareen*, Muhammad Al-Sweity, Wasef Alhroub, Kenana Altel and Abdalqader Aljaradat
Faculty of Medicine, Hebron University, Hebron, Palestine

*Address all correspondence to: maaweyajabreen6154572@gmail.com

References

[1] Jamil A, Mukkamalla SKR. Lymphoma. 2024

[2] Mugnaini EN, Ghosh N. Lymphoma. Primary Care Clinics in Office Practice. 2016;**43**:661-675. DOI: 10.1016/j.pop.2016.07.012

[3] Teras LR, DeSantis CE, Cerhan JR, et al. 2016 US lymphoid malignancy statistics by World Health Organization subtypes. CA: A Cancer Journal for Clinicians. 2016;**66**:443-459. DOI: 10.3322/caac.21357

[4] Matasar MJ, Zelenetz AD. Overview of lymphoma diagnosis and management. Radiologic Clinics of North America. 2008;**46**:175-198. DOI: 10.1016/j.rcl.2008.03.005

[5] Ansell SM. Hodgkin lymphoma: 2023 update on diagnosis, risk-stratification, and management. American Journal of Hematology. 2022;**97**:1478-1488. DOI: 10.1002/ajh.26717

[6] Shanbhag S, Ambinder RF. Hodgkin lymphoma: A review and update on recent progress. CA: A Cancer Journal for Clinicians. 2018;**68**:116-132. DOI: 10.3322/caac.21438

[7] Brice P, de Kerviler E, Friedberg JW. Classical Hodgkin lymphoma. Lancet. 2021;**398**:1518-1527. DOI: 10.1016/S0140-6736(20)32207-8

[8] Barrington SF, Kirkwood AA, Franceschetto A, et al. PET-CT for staging and early response: Results from the response-adapted therapy in advanced Hodgkin lymphoma study. Blood. 2016;**127**:1531-1538. DOI: 10.1182/blood-2015-11-679407

[9] Küppers R. New insights in the biology of Hodgkin lymphoma. Hematology. 2012;**2012**:328-334. DOI: 10.1182/asheducation.V2012.1.328.3798326

[10] Eichenauer DA, Engert A. How I treat nodular lymphocyte-predominant Hodgkin lymphoma. Blood. 2020;**136**:2987-2993. DOI: 10.1182/blood.2019004044

[11] Savage KJ, Mottok A, Fanale M. Nodular lymphocyte-predominant Hodgkin lymphoma. Seminars in Hematology. 2016;**53**:190-202. DOI: 10.1053/j.seminhematol.2016.05.009

[12] Sehn LH, Salles G. Diffuse large B-cell lymphoma. The New England Journal of Medicine. 2021;**384**:842-858. DOI: 10.1056/NEJMra2027612

[13] Sander B, Campo E, Hsi ED. Chronic lymphocytic leukaemia/small lymphocytic lymphoma and mantle cell lymphoma: From early lesions to transformation. Virchows Archiv. 2023;**482**:131-145. DOI: 10.1007/s00428-022-03460-y

[14] Parikh SA, Kay NE, Shanafelt TD. Monoclonal B-cell lymphocytosis: Update on diagnosis, clinical outcome, and counseling. Clinical Advances in Hematology & Oncology. 2013;**11**:720-729

[15] Gonzalez-Mancera MS, Lopategui J, Hoffman D, et al. B-cell prolymphocytic leukemia: An enduring bona fide entity. International Journal of Hematology. 2024;**120**:252-255. DOI: 10.1007/s12185-024-03774-4

[16] Mirandari A, Parker H, Ashton-Key M, et al. The genomic and molecular landscape of splenic marginal zone lymphoma, biological and clinical implications. Exploration of Targeted

Anti-tumor Therapy. 2024;**5**:877-901. DOI: 10.37349/etat.2024.00253

[17] Troussard X, Maître E, Paillassa J. Hairy cell leukemia 2024: Update on diagnosis, risk-stratification, and treatment-annual updates in hematological malignancies. American Journal of Hematology. 2024;**99**:679-696. DOI: 10.1002/ajh.27240

[18] Hairy cell leukemia. n.d

[19] Tizro P, Abdulbaki R, Aggarwal A, et al. In: Tutar Y, editor. Splenic B-Cell Lymphoma/Leukemia, Unclassifiable. Rijeka: IntechOpen; 2022. Ch. 4

[20] Yilmaz E, Chhina A, Nava VE, et al. A review on splenic diffuse red pulp small B-cell lymphoma. Current Oncology. 2021;**28**:5148-5154. DOI: 10.3390/curroncol28060431

[21] Splenic diffuse red pulp small B cell lymphoma. n.d

[22] Robak T. Hairy-cell leukemia variant: Recent view on diagnosis, biology and treatment. Cancer Treatment Reviews. 2011;**37**:3-10. DOI: 10.1016/j.ctrv.2010.05.003

[23] Wang W, Lin P. Lymphoplasmacytic lymphoma and Waldenström macroglobulinaemia: Clinicopathological features and differential diagnosis. Pathology. 2020;**52**:6-14. DOI: 10.1016/j.pathol.2019.09.009

[24] Lymphoplasmacytic lymphoma. n.d

[25] Amaador K, Peeters H, Minnema MC, et al. Monoclonal gammopathy of renal significance (MGRS) histopathologic classification, diagnostic workup, and therapeutic options. The Netherlands Journal of Medicine. 2019;**77**:243-254

[26] MGUS-IGM. n.d

[27] Wahner-Roedler DL, Kyle RA. Heavy chain diseases. Best Practice & Research. Clinical Haematology. 2005;**18**:729-746. DOI: 10.1016/j.beha.2005.01.029

[28] Baloda V, Wheeler SE, Murray DL, et al. Mu heavy chain disease with MYD88 L265P mutation: An unusual manifestation of lymphoplasmacytic lymphoma. Diagnostic Pathology. 2022;**17**:63. DOI: 10.1186/s13000-022-01244-1

[29] Alsharif R, Dunleavy K. Burkitt lymphoma and other high-grade B-cell lymphomas with or without MYC, BCL2, and/or BCL6 rearrangements. Hematology/Oncology Clinics of North America. 2019;**33**:587-596. DOI: 10.1016/j.hoc.2019.04.001

[30] Lue JK, Luttwak E, Rivas-Delgado A, et al. Limited stage high grade B-cell lymphoma with MYC, BCL2 and/or BCL6 rearrangements: BCL2 rearrangements drives the poor outcomes. Blood Cancer Journal. 2024;**14**:178. DOI: 10.1038/s41408-024-01148-x

[31] Miyamoto K, Kobayashi Y, Maeshima AM, et al. Clinicopathological prognostic factors of 24 patients with B-cell lymphoma, unclassifiable, with features intermediate between diffuse large B-cell lymphoma and Burkitt lymphoma. International Journal of Hematology. 2016;**103**:693-702. DOI: 10.1007/s12185-016-1989-z

[32] Gualco G, Natkunam Y, Bacchi CE. The spectrum of B-cell lymphoma, unclassifiable, with features intermediate between diffuse large B-cell lymphoma and classical Hodgkin lymphoma: A description of 10 cases. Modern Pathology: An Official Journal of the United States and Canadian Academy

of Pathology, Inc. 2012;**25**:661-674. DOI: 10.1038/modpathol.2011.200

[33] Ikeda T, Gion Y, Yoshino T, et al. A review of EBV-positive mucocutaneous ulcers focusing on clinical and pathological aspects. Journal of Clinical and Experimental Hematopathology. 2019;**59**:64-71. DOI: 10.3960/jslrt.18039

[34] Tralongo P, Bakacs A, Larocca LM. EBV-related lymphoproliferative diseases: A review in light of new classifications. Mediterranean Journal of Hematology and Infectious Diseases. 2024;**16**:e2024042. DOI: 10.4084/MJHID.2024.042

[35] Swerdlow SH, Campo E, Pileri SA, et al. The 2016 revision of the World Health Organization classification of lymphoid neoplasms. Blood. 2016;**127**:2375-2390. DOI: 10.1182/blood-2016-01-643569

[36] Marcelis L, Tousseyn T, Sagaert X. MALT lymphoma as a model of chronic inflammation-induced gastric tumor development. 2019:77-106

[37] Fakhruddin N, Abou Dalle I, Chakhachiro Z. Primary mediastinal large B-cell lymphoma from the clinic to genomics: Insights for pathologists. Human Pathology. 2024:105705. DOI: 10.1016/j.humpath.2024.105705

[38] Nishii-Ito S, Izumi H, Touge H, et al. Pulmonary intravascular large B-cell lymphoma successfully treated with rituximab, cyclophosphamide, vincristine, doxorubicin and prednisolone immunochemotherapy: Report of a patient surviving for over 1 year. Molecular and Clinical Oncology. 2016;**5**:689-692. DOI: 10.3892/mco.2016.1063

[39] Baker J, Zadeh SL, Aguilera NS. ALK-positive large B-cell lymphoma (ALK + LBCL) with aberrant CD3 expression. Journal of Hematopathology. 2024;**17**:109-114. DOI: 10.1007/s12308-024-00582-x

[40] Morscio J, Dierickx D, Nijs J, et al. Clinicopathologic comparison of plasmablastic lymphoma in HIV-positive, immunocompetent, and posttransplant patients. The American Journal of Surgical Pathology. 2014;**38**:875-886. DOI: 10.1097/PAS.0000000000000234

[41] López de Cáceres CVB, Sant'Ana MSP, Roman Tager EMJ, et al. Extracavitary primary effusion lymphoma affecting the oral cavity: A rare case report. International Journal of Surgical Pathology. 2024;**32**:119-132. DOI: 10.1177/10668969231167509

[42] Castillo JJ, Beltran BE, Miranda RN, et al. EBV-positive diffuse large B-cell lymphoma, not otherwise specified: 2018 update on diagnosis, risk-stratification and management. American Journal of Hematology. 2018;**93**:953-962. DOI: 10.1002/ajh.25112

[43] Fang H, Wang W, Medeiros LJ. Burkitt lymphoma. Human Pathology. 2024:105703. DOI: 10.1016/j.humpath.2024.105703

[44] Wang Y, Chen D, Hu R, et al. Clinicopathological characteristics of light and heavy chain deposition disease: A case series. American Journal of Kidney Diseases. 2024;**84**:447-456.e1. DOI: 10.1053/j.ajkd.2024.03.021

[45] Zhang Y, Li X, Liang D, et al. Heavy chain deposition disease: Clinicopathologic characteristics of a Chinese case series. American Journal of Kidney Diseases. 2020;**75**:736-743. DOI: 10.1053/j.ajkd.2019.08.013

[46] Campo E, Jaffe ES, Cook JR, et al. The international consensus

classification of mature lymphoid neoplasms: A report from the clinical advisory committee. Blood. 2022;**140**:1229-1253. DOI: 10.1182/blood.2022015851

[47] Weinhold N, Johnson DC, Rawstron AC, et al. Inherited genetic susceptibility to monoclonal gammopathy of unknown significance. Blood. 2014;**123**:2513-2517. DOI: 10.1182/blood-2013-10-532283

[48] Siegel RL, Miller KD, Fuchs HE, et al. Cancer statistics, 2021. CA: A Cancer Journal for Clinicians. 2021;**71**:7-33. DOI: 10.3322/caac.21654

[49] Rajkumar SV. Multiple myeloma: 2024 update on diagnosis, risk-stratification, and management. American Journal of Hematology. 2024;**99**:1802-1824. DOI: 10.1002/ajh.27422

[50] Nahi H, Genell A, Wålinder G, et al. Incidence, characteristics, and outcome of solitary plasmacytoma and plasma cell leukemia. Population-based data from the Swedish myeloma register. European Journal of Haematology. 2017;**99**:216-222. DOI: 10.1111/ejh.12907

[51] Ozsahin M, Tsang RW, Poortmans P, et al. Outcomes and patterns of failure in solitary plasmacytoma: A multicenter rare cancer network study of 258 patients. International Journal of Radiation Oncology, Biology, Physics. 2006;**64**:210-217. DOI: 10.1016/j.ijrobp.2005.06.039

[52] Jaafar NA, Hussain FA, Mat Lazim N. Successful treatment of extraosseous plasmacytoma of the oropharynx with cervical lymph node involvement. Indian Journal of Otolaryngology and Head and Neck Surgery: Official Publication of the Association of Otolaryngologists of India. 2024;**76**:1220-1223. DOI: 10.1007/s12070-023-04228-9

[53] Zucca E, Bertoni F. The spectrum of MALT lymphoma at different sites: Biological and therapeutic relevance. Blood. 2016;**127**:2082-2092. DOI: 10.1182/blood-2015-12-624304

[54] Da B, Zhang J, Zhu F, et al. Extranodal marginal zone lymphoma of mucosa-associated lymphoid tissue of the ileum in an adult presenting with intussusception: A case report and literature review. Frontiers in Oncology. 2024;**14**. DOI: 10.3389/fonc.2024.1395144

[55] Hori D, Kobayashi R, Suzuki D, et al. Pediatric nodal marginal zone lymphoma in a Japanese boy. Pediatrics International. 2017;**59**:358-360. DOI: 10.1111/ped.13188

[56] Attarbaschi A, Abla O, Arias Padilla L, et al. Rare non-Hodgkin lymphoma of childhood and adolescence: A consensus diagnostic and therapeutic approach to pediatric-type follicular lymphoma, marginal zone lymphoma, and nonanaplastic peripheral T-cell lymphoma. Pediatric Blood & Cancer. 2020;**67**:e28416. DOI: 10.1002/pbc.28416

[57] Schmidt J, Ramis-Zaldivar JE, Bonzheim I, et al. CREBBP gene mutations are frequently detected in in situ follicular neoplasia. Blood. 2018;**132**:2687-2690

[58] Kurz KS, Kalmbach S, Ott M, et al. Follicular lymphoma in the 5th edition of the WHO-classification of haematolymphoid neoplasms-updated classification and new biological data. Cancers (Basel). 2023;**15**. DOI: 10.3390/cancers15030785

[59] Agostinelli C, Akarca AU, Ramsay A, et al. Novel markers in pediatric-type follicular lymphoma. Virchows Archiv. 2019;**475**:771-779. DOI: 10.1007/s00428-019-02681-y

[60] Pizzi M, Bongiovanni L, Lorenzi L, et al. Large B-cell lymphoma with IRF4 rearrangement: A multi-centric study with focus on potential misleading phenotypes. Virchows Archiv. 2024;**484**:521-526. DOI: 10.1007/s00428-023-03689-1

[61] Kim DH, Li S, Garces S, et al. Large B-cell lymphoma with IRF4 rearrangement and follicular pattern: A differential diagnosis of follicular lymphoma. Human Pathology Reports. 2022;**27**:300602. DOI: 10.1016/j.hpr.2022.300602

[62] Specht L, Dabaja B, Illidge T, et al. Modern radiation therapy for primary cutaneous lymphomas: Field and dose guidelines from the international lymphoma radiation oncology group. International Journal of Radiation Oncology, Biology, Physics. 2015;**92**:32-39. DOI: 10.1016/j.ijrobp.2015.01.008

[63] Baermann B-N, Dietrich S. Mantle cell lymphoma. In: The EBMT Handbook. Cham: Springer International Publishing; 2024. pp. 787-790

[64] Oishi N, Montes-Moreno S, Feldman AL. In situ neoplasia in lymph node pathology. Seminars in Diagnostic Pathology. 2018;**35**:76-83. DOI: 10.1053/j.semdp.2017.11.001

[65] Laurini JA, Perry AM, Boilesen E, et al. Classification of non-Hodgkin lymphoma in central and South America: A review of 1028 cases. Blood. 2012;**120**:4795-4801. DOI: 10.1182/blood-2012-07-440073

[66] Toumi A, Fazal S, Litaiem N. Lymphomatoid Papulosis. 2025

[67] Baik BS, Lee WS, Ji SY, et al. Treatment of primary cutaneous anaplastic large cell lymphoma. Archives of Craniofacial Surgery. 2019;**20**:207-211. DOI: 10.7181/acfs.2018.02201

[68] Goyal A, Goyal K, Bohjanen K, et al. Epidemiology of primary cutaneous γδ T-cell lymphoma and subcutaneous panniculitis-like T-cell lymphoma in the U.S.A. from 2006 to 2015: A surveillance, epidemiology, and end results-18 analysis. The British Journal of Dermatology. 2019;**181**:848-850. DOI: 10.1111/bjd.17985

[69] Salaverria I, Martin-Guerrero I, Wagener R, et al. A recurrent 11q aberration pattern characterizes a subset of MYC-negative high-grade B-cell lymphomas resembling Burkitt lymphoma. Blood. 2014;**123**:1187-1198. DOI: 10.1182/blood-2013-06-507996

[70] Gutierrez M, Bladek P, Goksu B, et al. T-cell prolymphocytic Leukemia: Diagnosis, pathogenesis, and treatment. International Journal of Molecular Sciences. 2023;**24**. DOI: 10.3390/ijms241512106

[71] Park SH, Lee YJ, Kim Y, et al. T-large granular lymphocytic leukemia. Blood Research. 2023;**58**:S52-S57. DOI: 10.5045/br.2023.2023037

[72] Poullot E, Zambello R, Leblanc F, et al. Chronic natural killer lymphoproliferative disorders: Characteristics of an international cohort of 70 patients. Annals of Oncology. 2014;**25**:2030-2035. DOI: 10.1093/annonc/mdu369

[73] Sumbly V, Vest M, Landry I. Aggressive natural killer cell leukemia: A brief overview of its genomic landscape, histological features, and current management. Cureus. 2022;**14**:e22537. DOI: 10.7759/cureus.22537

[74] Tabanelli V, Agostinelli C, Sabattini E, et al. Systemic Epstein-Barr-virus-positive T cell lymphoproliferative childhood disease in a 22-year-old Caucasian man: A case report and

review of the literature. Journal of Medical Case Reports. 2011;**5**:218. DOI: 10.1186/1752-1947-5-218

[75] Wang X, Liang Y, Yang Y, et al. Hydroa vacciniforme-like lymphoproliferative disorder: A clinicopathological, immunohistochemical, and prognostic study of 24 cases in China. The Journal of Dermatology. 2021;**48**:1315-1326. DOI: 10.1111/1346-8138.15944

[76] Durer C, Babiker HM. Adult T-Cell Leukemia. Treasure Island (FL); 2025

[77] Shah UA, Shah N, Qiao B, et al. Epidemiology and survival trend of adult T-cell leukemia/lymphoma in the United States. Cancer. 2020;**126**:567-574. DOI: 10.1002/cncr.32556

[78] Sánchez-Romero C, Bologna-Molina R, Paes de Almeida O, et al. Extranodal NK/T cell lymphoma, nasal type: An updated overview. Critical Reviews in Oncology/Hematology. 2021;**159**:103237. DOI: 10.1016/j.critrevonc.2021.103237

[79] Al Somali Z, Hamadani M, Kharfan-Dabaja M, et al. Enteropathy-associated T cell lymphoma. Current Hematologic Malignancy Reports. 2021;**16**:140-147. DOI: 10.1007/s11899-021-00634-4

[80] Zhou B, Guo M, Li X, et al. Clinicopathological and molecular genetic alterations in monomorphic–epitheliotropic intestinal T-cell lymphoma of the small intestine. European Journal of Medical Research. 2024;**29**:191. DOI: 10.1186/s40001-024-01797-5

[81] Fan W, Niu L, He H, et al. Indolent T-cell lymphoproliferative disorder of gastrointestinal tract with unusual clinical courses: Report of 6 cases and literature review. Virchows Archiv. 2023;**482**:729-743. DOI: 10.1007/s00428-022-03467-5

[82] Chowdhury Z, Khonglah Y, Raphael V, et al. Hepatosplenic T cell lymphoma: Diagnostic conundrum. International Journal of Hematology-oncology and Stem Cell Research. 2022;**16**:66-73

[83] Rahman K, Gupta T, Gupta R, et al. Hepatosplenic T-cell lymphoma diagnosed using flow cytometry. A single-center study of 12 cases from North India. Journal of Cancer Research and Therapeutics. 2022;**18**:1093-1097. DOI: 10.4103/jcrt.JCRT_877_19

[84] Musick SR, Lynch DT. Subcutaneous Panniculitis-like T-Cell Lymphoma. Treasure Island (FL); 2025

[85] Fort C, Raina R, Surapaneni R. An institutional experience of a rare diagnosis of subcutaneous panniculitis-like T-cell lymphoma. Journal of Clinical Oncology. 2024;**42**:e19073. DOI: 10.1200/JCO.2024.42.16_suppl.e19073

[86] Lee H. Mycosis fungoides and Sézary syndrome. Blood Research. 2023;**58**:S66-S82. DOI: 10.5045/br.2023.2023023

[87] García-Díaz N, Piris MÁ, Ortiz-Romero PL, et al. Mycosis fungoides and Sézary syndrome: An integrative review of the pathophysiology, molecular drivers, and targeted therapy. Cancers (Basel). 2021;**13**. DOI: 10.3390/cancers13081931

[88] Beltraminelli H, Leinweber B, Kerl H, et al. Primary cutaneous CD4+ small–/medium-sized pleomorphic T-cell lymphoma: A cutaneous nodular proliferation of pleomorphic T lymphocytes of undetermined significance? A study of 136 cases. The American Journal of Dermatopathology. 2009;**31**:317-322. DOI: 10.1097/DAD.0b013e31819f19bb

[89] Broccoli A, Zinzani PL. Peripheral T-cell lymphoma, not otherwise specified. Blood. 2017;**129**:1103-1112. DOI: 10.1182/blood-2016-08-692566

[90] Project IT-CL. International peripheral T-cell and natural killer/T-cell lymphoma study: Pathology findings and clinical outcomes. Journal of Clinical Oncology. 2008;**26**:4124-4130

[91] Ree HJ, Kadin ME, Kikuchi M, et al. Angioimmunoblastic lymphoma (AILD-type T-cell lymphoma) with hyperplastic germinal centers. The American Journal of Surgical Pathology. 1998;**22**

[92] Weisenburger DD, Savage KJ, Harris NL, et al. Peripheral T-cell lymphoma, not otherwise specified: A report of 340 cases from the international peripheral T-cell lymphoma project. Blood. 2011;**117**:3402-3408. DOI: 10.1182/blood-2010-09-310342

[93] Alaggio R, Amador C, Anagnostopoulos I, et al. The 5th edition of the World Health Organization classification of haematolymphoid tumours: Lymphoid neoplasms. Leukemia. 2022;**36**:1720-1748. DOI: 10.1038/s41375-022-01620-2

[94] Fujisawa M, Sakata-Yanagimoto M, Nishizawa S, et al. Activation of RHOA-VAV1 signaling in angioimmunoblastic T-cell lymphoma. Leukemia. 2018;**32**:694-702. DOI: 10.1038/leu.2017.273

[95] Tsuyama N, Sakamoto K, Sakata S, et al. Anaplastic large cell lymphoma: Pathology, genetics, and clinical aspects. Journal of Clinical and Experimental Hematopathology. 2017;**57**:120-142. DOI: 10.3960/jslrt.17023

[96] Savage KJ, Harris NL, Vose JM, et al. ALK−anaplastic large-cell lymphoma is clinically and immunophenotypically different from both ALK+ ALCL and peripheral T-cell lymphoma, not otherwise specified: Report from the international peripheral T-cell lymphoma project. Blood, J Am Soc Hematol. 2008;**111**:5496-5504

[97] Quesada AE, Medeiros LJ, Clemens MW, et al. Breast implant-associated anaplastic large cell lymphoma: A review. Modern Pathology: An Official Journal of the United States and Canadian Academy of Pathology, Inc. 2019;**32**:166-188. DOI: 10.1038/s41379-018-0134-3

[98] Sapkota S, Shaikh H. Non-Hodgkin Lymphoma. 2024

[99] Eichenauer DA, Aleman BMP, André M, et al. Hodgkin lymphoma: ESMO clinical practice guidelines for diagnosis, treatment and follow-up. Annals of Oncology. 2018;**29**:iv19-iv29. DOI: 10.1093/annonc/mdy080

[100] Lewis WD, Lilly S, Jones KL. Lymphoma: Diagnosis and treatment. American Family Physician. 2020;**101**:34-41. DOI: 31894937

[101] Coiffier B, Thieblemont C, Van Den Neste E, et al. Long-term outcome of patients in the LNH-98.5 trial, the first randomized study comparing rituximab-CHOP to standard CHOP chemotherapy in DLBCL patients: A study by the Groupe d'Etudes des Lymphomes de l'Adulte. Blood. 2010;**116**:2040-2045. DOI: 10.1182/blood-2010-03-276246

[102] Hoppe RT, Advani RH, Ai WZ, et al. NCCN guidelines® insights: Hodgkin lymphoma, version 2.2022. Journal of the National Comprehensive Cancer Network. 2022;**20**:322-334. DOI: 10.6004/jnccn.2022.0021

[103] Perales M-A, Ceberio I, Armand P, et al. Role of cytotoxic therapy with

hematopoietic cell transplantation in the treatment of Hodgkin lymphoma: Guidelines from the American Society for Blood and Marrow Transplantation. Biology of Blood and Marrow Transplantation. 2015;**21**:971-983. DOI: 10.1016/j.bbmt.2015.02.022

[104] Vassilakopoulos TP, Asimakopoulos JV, Konstantopoulos K, et al. Optimizing outcomes in relapsed/refractory Hodgkin lymphoma: A review of current and forthcoming therapeutic strategies. Therapeutic Advances in Hematology. 2020;**11**. DOI: 10.1177/2040620720902911

[105] Sharma P, Allison JP. The future of immune checkpoint therapy. Science. 2015;**348**:56-61. DOI: 10.1126/science.aaa8172

Chapter 6

Castleman Disease

Prakash Sivaramakrishnan

Abstract

Castleman disease (CD) is a rare, nonclonal lymphoproliferative disorder with varied clinical and pathological manifestations and often mimics malignancies or infections like tuberculosis. It is broadly classified into *unicentric (UCD)* and *multicentric (MCD)* forms, with MCD further subdivided into *HHV-8–associated, idiopathic (iMCD)*, and *TAFRO syndrome*. The primary pathogenetic mechanism involves *cytokine dysregulation (IL-6, VEGF)*, but can also include viral triggers (HHV-8) and genetic mutations. Diagnosis relies on *histopathology* (hyaline vascular or plasma cell variants) and exclusion of mimics such as lymphoma, TB. *Imaging (CT/MRI/PET)* aids in localization, guides biopsy, and serves as a prognostic marker in CD. *IL-6 blockade (siltuximab)* is first line for iMCD. *UCD has excellent prognosis with surgery*, whereas *MCD requires systemic therapy* and has a relapse risk. Poor prognostic markers include anemia, hypoalbuminemia, and organomegaly. Collaborative research is critical to unravel CD's complexity and improve outcomes.

Keywords: Castleman disease, HHV-8-negative multicentric castleman, interleukin-6 (IL-6) blockade, lymphoproliferative disorders, Tafro syndrome

1. Introduction

Castleman disease (CD) is a nonclonal lymphoproliferative disorder which is often considered as a rare cause of nonneoplastic lymphadenopathy. Its manifestations can be diverse owing to its ability to affect all organs. Due to the manifestation being mediastinal lymph node enlargement, it is considered as an eternal mimic to innumerous benign and malignant diseases such as lymphomas, cancers, and tuberculosis. It is broadly divided into unicentric Castleman disease (UCD) and multicentric Castleman disease (MCD). In general, an astute clinician should suspect Castleman disease in any patient presenting with a hyperenhancing lymph nodal mass. Castleman is as similar to sarcoidosis in being a disease of exclusion, which imperatively suggests that it must be considered in the differential diagnosis of lymphoma, metastatic lymphadenopathy, and ubiquitous diseases that result in adenopathy like tuberculosis and sarcoidosis.

In recent times, research into Castleman disease has resulted in division of CD into a spectrum of pathologic variants, including the classic hyaline vascular type, plasma cell variant of Castleman disease, and the multicentric Castleman disease. Multicentric Castleman disease is further divided into multiple sub-types which is described in detail in this chapter.

Castleman disease is known to be associated with a wide host of conditions, most common among which include human immunodeficiency virus, lymphoma, thrombocytopenia, anasarca, fever/elevated C-reactive protein (CRP), renal dysfunction/reticulin myelofibrosis, organomegaly (TAFRO), POEMS syndrome (polyneuropathy, organomegaly, endocrinopathy, M protein, and skin changes), paraneoplastic pemphigus, and plasma cell dyscrasias. CD patients are usually asymptomatic, and abnormalities on imaging are incidentally detected, with clinical spectrum varying from asymptomatic lymphadenopathy to aggressive forms threatening organ failure. Unicentric Castleman disease is often curable with surgery/localized radiation therapy, whereas multicentric Castleman disease warrants longer treatment durations with chemotherapy anti IL-6 therapy, and local radiation therapy, or the use of monoclonal antibodies. Relapses or recurrences are also documents in cases of Castleman disease. This chapter focusses briefly on Castleman disease, its history, epidemiology, pathology, clinical presentation, and its management.

2. History of Castleman disease

Castleman disease (CD) was first described by Benjamin Castleman and Virginia Towne in the year 1954 at the clinicopathological conference of the Massachusetts General Hospital [1, 2]. The first description was of a patient having unicentric Castleman disease. During the first description by Castleman and Towne, they also went on to present 12 additional cases with similar histopathological findings. Similar case findings were also reported by Flendrig [3] and Schillings in 1969 and by Keller et al. [4] in 1972, and two variants were identified, both of which presented as distinct mass lesions. One subtype was the hyaline vascular type which was described as having prominent hyalinization, regressive follicles, and increased vascularity, whereas the second type was a plasma cell type dominated by plasma cells and usually presents with systemic symptoms.

The next breakthrough in CD occurred in 1980, when Glauco Frizzera and Juan Rosai described ten patients with a multicentric lymphoid disorder with histological features resembling UCD with systemic features.

The first description of HHV-associated multicentric Castleman disease was put forth in 1984 by Chang et al. [5]. In this case report, HHV8 (KSHV) was first isolated from a patient with HIV and suspected Kaposi sarcoma. Subsequently, it was determined to be a causative factor for the development of Castleman disease, which has led to advancement in understanding of the pathogenesis of Castleman disease.

3. Epidemiology of Castleman disease

3.1 Unicentric Castleman disease

The International Classification of Diseases (ICD) classification for Castleman disease became effective on October 1, 2016, under the code ICD-10-CM-D47.Z2. However, till this time, no formal definition was available, which is one of the reasons for inaccurate assessment of the epidemiology of this disease. Since publication of this criteria in the ICD-10, more cases are being reported, and a consensus diagnostic criterion has been made for CD [6].

Unicentric Castleman disease can manifest at all ages, but it peaks at a younger age, more precisely the 3rd and 4th decade. Also, unicentric CD is known to present at an earlier age in comparison with multicentric CD. Further details regarding age of onset of various subtypes of CD are shown in **Table 1**.

DOI: http://dx.doi.org/10.5772/intechopen.1009424

	Hyaline vascular CD	**Plasma cell CD**	**HHV-8 associated CD**	**iMCD TAFRO**	**iMCD, NOS (includes multiple subtypes)**
Clinical Features	Young adults (mediantthird-fourth decade)	Localized—3rd/ 4th decade Generalized—Elderly	Immunosuppressed and/or HIV-positive patients	Rapid deterioration and serious disease.	Age variable (median sixth decade)
Presentation	UCD > MCD	MCD > UCD Generally associated with Fever Loss of wright, Night sweats	Diffuse lymph nodal enlargement, Fever Loss of weight/appetite Immune abnormalities (likely associated with HIV)	TAFRO	Generalized LAD, constitutional symptoms, hematologic and/or immunologic abnormalities
Probable pathogenic factors	Unknown VEGF FDC's predominance	IL-6	HHV-8	Cytokine storm and Hyper IL-6 syndrome	IL-6, Genetic mechanisms, Polymorphisms
Associated lesions	Follicular dendritic cell neoplasms, vascular/ stromal neoplasms, plasmacytoid dendritic cell collections	POEMS syndrome, Plasma cell aggregations (usually single type of cells)	Lymphoma (plasmablastic and KSHV associated lymphoproliferative disease, Kaposi sarcoma)	Thrombocytopenia, anasarca, edema, pleural effusion, and ascites, fever, reticulin myelofibrosis	Similar to plasma cell CD, also associated with increased risk of other lymphomas

Table 1.
Features of various subtypes of Castleman disease.

UCD is a rare disease, and no authentic data is available regarding its incidence. However, extrapolations have been made from insurance databases of various countries. Varying incidences have been reported from different countries, with a study from China reporting the incidence at 16 per million [7, 8]. Other data is reported from case reports and case series, but there is an inherent risk of bias in these reports due to the fact that they have all been reported from tertiary or centers of excellence. A significant majority of patients are known to have HV type of UCD, and although the cause remains unclear, there is evidence that it is a clonal disease.

3.2 Multicentric Castleman disease

3.2.1 HHV-8 MCD

HHV-8 was first described by Chang et al. in 1994 [5, 9]. Chang and associates extracted herpesvirus-like DNA sequences from Kaposi sarcoma lesions in AIDS patients, which led to the discovery of HHV-8. The seroprevalence ranges from 2 to 4% in the Caribbean, Southeast Asia, and northern Europe. Prevalence rates are highest in sub-Saharan Africa at over 40%, whereas rates are greater in Mediterranean populations (i.e., Israel, Saudi Arabia, Italy, and Greece) at about 10%.

3.2.2 iMCD

The cause of iMCD is uncertain [10]. Some hypothesized mechanisms include secretion of paracrine cytokines by neoplastic cells when infected with a virus other than HHV-8. This can also happen as a result of autoinflammatory processes or genetic abnormalities in the control of IL-6. Because this CD subgroup is more diverse than the others, it is possible—indeed, likely—that there are multiple causes. HIV-negative MCD was estimated to be 5 per million based on data from an insurance database.

3.2.3 MCD-TAFRO

In 2010, it was initially reported in a set of Japanese subjects [11, 12]. Data about its incidence is quite scarce. Only 1 individual (1.3%) met the TAFRO diagnostic criteria in a Beijing series that included 144 cases of CD, including 79 with MCD. A series from MD Anderson, on the other hand, reported a 21% incidence of TAFRO, which may have been the result of referral bias. Geographically, the incidence may vary, although it may be around 2% of iMCD cases.

4. Pathogenesis of Castleman disease

Although the exact origin of CD is still unknown, Yoshizaki et al. [13] suggest that the pathophysiology of CD may be influenced by four primary factors: cytokine imbalances, viral infections, immune system dysfunction, and genetic abnormalities (**Figure 1**).

In this section, we will discuss briefly discuss regarding the pathogenetic mechanisms for the disease initiation and progression among CD patients. In depth molecular description regarding the pathogenesis is out of the scope of this chapter, and the reader is advised to refer to literature referenced in bibliography for further reading.

Cytokine imbalance [14, 15]: Studies indicate that in a sizable portion of patients, interleukin-6 (IL-6) is the primary starter and most important factor in the

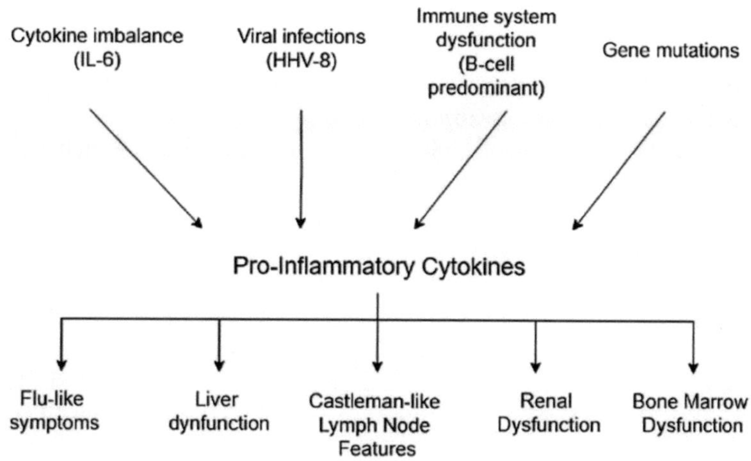

Figure 1.
Pathogenetic mechanisms of development of Castleman disease.

pathophysiology of CD. One significant contributing cause to the aberrant proliferation of plasma cells in lymphoid organs is IL-6.

It activates the following pathways

- Janus kinase/signal transducer and activator of transcription (JAK/STAT)
- Ras-mitogen-activated protein kinase (MAPK)
- p38
- c-Jun N-terminal kinase (JNK)
- MAPK
- phosphoinositide 3-kinase/Akt/mammalian target of rapamycin (PI3K/Akt/mTOR)
- MEK-ERK5 pathways.

This increased secretion is enhanced in CD31 secreting cells, suggesting vasculogenic hypothesis for IL-6 production. But, in spite of this central role played by IL-6, a substantial minority of patients do not respond to IL-6 therapies, thus suggesting plausible other cells/cytokines in the pathogenesis of CD.

Other cytokines and factors include

- Vascular endothelial growth factor (VEGF) [16, 17] promotes angiogenesis (more in iMCD and POEMS-MCD)
- Chemokine ligand 13 (CXCL13: It is an important cytokine responsible for the pathogenesis of CD. In addition, CXCL13 is also used as a biomarker for predicting the response of iMCD to siltuximab.)
- IL-1β: Interleukin-1 beta (IL-1β).

4.1 Viral infection

Uncontrolled HHV-8 infection is a known etiological driver of HHV-8-related MCD [16–20]. HHV-8 is linked to abnormal cytokine regulation, and this hypothesis was confirmed by the detection of high levels of human IL-6 and human IL-10 in patient serum during active MCD episodes.

4.2 Immune system dysfunction

One of the mechanisms underlying the onset of CD may be abnormal immune cell activation, particularly of B cells [17–19]. CD development is also linked to peripheral T cells, including the polyfunctional effector memory CD8 + T cells. A study revealed that a decreased CD4/CD8 ratio was present in 32% of CD cases across all spectrum.

4.3 Gene mutations

Previously, CD was considered a disease of hyperplasia of lymph nodes [20–24]. But a wide array of genetic markers are known to be associated with development of CD. They are enumerated below.

- CXCL13.
- Enhanced expression of angiogenesis factors (e.g., LPL, DLL4)
- Extracellular matrix remodeling factors (including TGFβ, SKIL, LOXL1, IL-1β, ADAM33, and CLEC4A)
- Components of the complement system (C3, CR2)
- Markers indicative of germinal center activation (ZDHHC2 and BLK)
- Upregulation of IL-6 signaling components (IL-6 signal transducer, oncostatin M receptor, and leukemia inhibitory factor receptor),
- IL-2
- Markers of plasma cell differentiation (XBP1),
- Cytokines associated with fibroblastic reticular cells (CCL21),
- VEGF
- Mechanistic target of rapamycin complex 1 pathway.

5. Pathology of Castleman disease

5.1 Unicentric Castleman disease

The two main categories of histologic findings in UCD are follicular changes and interfollicular/stromal changes [4, 25].

Increased follicle count, dispersed across the cortex and medulla, and the presence of two or more tiny germinal centers (also known as twinning) are characteristics of follicular alterations.

- HV lesions, sometimes referred to as lollipop lesions, are created when sclerotic blood vessels radially penetrate the germinal centers.

- These follicles have wide mantle zones, which are frequently made up of concentric rings of tiny lymphocytes (also known as the "onion skin pattern").

Several high endothelial venules with plump endothelial cells make up the interfollicular areas in HV-CD, and sclerotic walls are common in vessels. The interfollicular regions frequently (though not always) contain clusters of plasmacytoid dendritic cells, which typically have a starry sky pattern.

Having follicles that make up more than 50% of the lymph node is an arbitrary definition of follicular HV-CD. Many sclerotic blood arteries and other spindle cells can subtotally replace the lymph node in the stroma-rich types of HV-CD, where interfollicular abnormalities make up over 50% of the lymph node.

These interfollicular regions have been called angiomyoid, histiocytic reticulum cell, or FDC stromal proliferations according to their varying cell makeup as assessed by immunohistochemistry reactivity for actin, CD68, or dendritic cell markers.

When making a diagnosis, it is crucial to rule out multicentric CD because unicentric PC-CD is less common, particularly in patients with systemic symptoms.

In unicentric PC-CD, sheets of mature PCs, with sporadic binucleated forms, occupy the medulla and interfollicular regions.

Despite the occurrence of light chain restricted PCs in rare instances, the PCs are polytypic by immunohistochemical evaluation for kappa and lambda. In the interfollicular spaces, vascular growth varies.

5.2 Multicentric Castleman disease

Regardless of the cause, all multicentric CD patients have similar morphologic characteristics [25–27].

Although lymphoid follicles can be hyperplastic, a subset of them frequently exhibit certain HV abnormalities, such as mantle zones that resemble onion peel and tiny germinal centers with lymphocyte depletion. The radial arteriole that penetrates the germinal center typically lacks sclerotic walls, in contrast to HV-CD.

Kaposi sarcoma and HHV8-diffuse large B-cell lymphoma are two HHV8-associated neoplasms that are more likely to coexist in patients with HHV8 multicentric CD.

Lymph nodes in TAFRO patients have a combination of traits from PC and HV variants, enlarged reticulin fibrosis, and enlarged megakaryocytes that may exhibit split nuclear lobes, and occasionally emperipolesis are all visible in the bone marrow of patients with TAFRO.

While some HV follicles may be present, the majority of CD instances in POEMS syndrome exhibit characteristics of the PC variety.

5.3 Immunohistochemistry

A host of IHC markers can be positive in Castleman disease [28, 29]. It depends on the area and the type of tissue which is usually stained.

1. Follicular dendritic cells: CD21, CD23, CD35, and epidermal growth factor receptor

2. Dendritic cells. They are usually positive for vascular cell adhesion molecule (VCAM-1, CD106).

3. B cells: CD10 and BCL-6 and negative for BCL-2

4. Mantle zones of the follicles: polytypic light chains, CD19, CD20, IgD, and BCL-2 are negative for CD10 and BCL-6.

In HV-CD—IL-6 staining is usually negative, whereas in PC-CD and MCD—IL-6 staining is usually positive owing to its unique pathogenetic mechanism.

HHV8 and EBV tests are often negative in PC-CD. Monoclonal antibodies that are specific to viral components can be used to demonstrate the virus in HHV8 multicentric CD. The most utilized antibody is a commercially available antibody specific to latent nuclear antigen (LANA-1).

Plasma cells are typically polytypic in HHV8 and HHV8-negative forms of multicentric CD. IgM1 cells are more prevalent around follicles, while IgG1 and IgA1 cells are primarily seen in the interfollicular regions. The PCs express a variety of heavy chains. However, the PCs may be monotypic in as many as one-third of multicentric CD cases. The PCs nearly invariably express both IgG or IgA and cytoplasmic lambda when they are monotypic. When HHV8 or POEMS syndrome is present, monotypic PCs are more common.

Molecular Analysis [29, 30]: Gene alterations are most seen in HHV-8 positive MCD (HIV-associated).

Genetic translocations have also been known in patients with CD, and they are listed below:

- t(1;16) (p11;p11)
- t(1;22) (p22;q13)
- t(7;8) (qter;q12)
- High mobility group protein isoform C (HMGIC)
- Human androgen receptor alpha (HUMARA)
- IL-6 loci - t(7;14) (p22;q22)
- T-cell receptor gene rearrangements are rare in multicentric CD, in less than 10% of cases.

6. Subtypes and classification

Castleman disease is a benign lymphoproliferative disease that has the propensity to occur all throughout the body [31]. An approximate 70% of Castleman disease occurs in the thoracic cavity, with involvement of the neck in about 15% patients, and an approximate 15% show involvement of the abdomen and pelvis. Irrespective of the region of involvement, it predominantly involves the primary lymphatic tissues. On occasion, involvement of the extralymphatic sites can be seen which include parotid glands, pancreas, meninges, liver, and the laryngeal tissues.

Historically, Castleman disease has been classified in two broad classifications

a. Morphological

b. Histopathological and genetic.

Morphological classification is either unicentric or multicentric, which is decided on the basis of extensiveness of lymphadenopathy.

Histopathological classification is based on the pathological variations on tissue specimens. The spectrum of Castleman disease is depicted in **Figure 2**. Subtypes of Castleman disease are given in **Figure 2**. Various features of the different subtypes are shown in **Table 1**.

Hyaline vascular Castleman disease, plasma cell Castleman disease, human herpesvirus 8 (HHV-8)-associated Castleman disease, and multicentric Castleman disease not otherwise defined are the several types of Castleman disease that are distinguished by the histological classification.

Unicentric Castleman disease has mainly two types, namely the hyaline vascular (HV-CD), and the plasma cell variant (PC-CD). Multicentric Castleman disease is further classified as HHV-8 positive and HHV-8 negative disease. HHV-8 is subclassified into other variants based on the microscopic and molecular tests of histopathological examination. The last piece of the classification puzzle is the Idiopathic MCD, which is not a clearly distinct group is closely associated to the historical classification of Castleman disease into unicentric and multicentric Castleman disease.

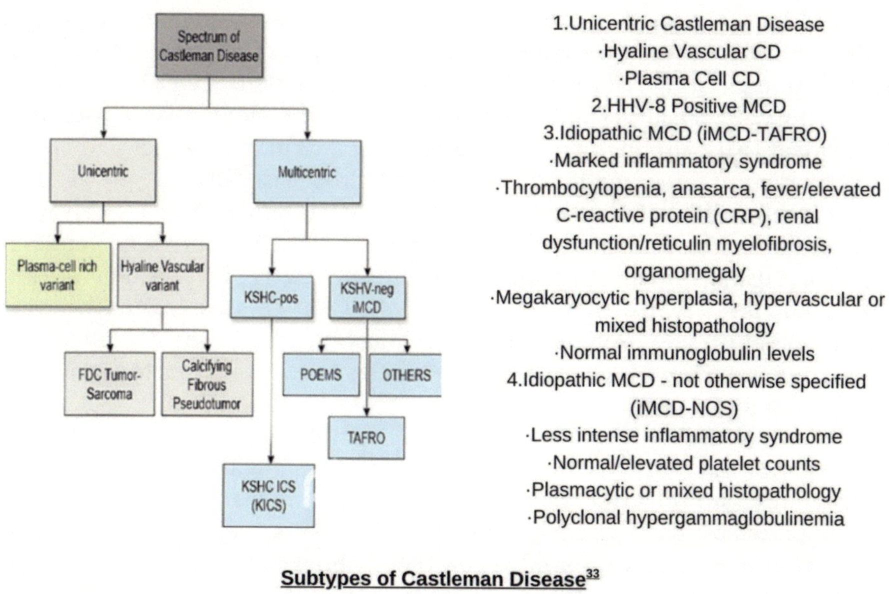

Figure 2.
Spectrum and subtypes of Castleman disease.

It is further subdivided into other pathological variants based on the association with HHV-8 and the morphological resemblance to the variants of UCD which are PC-CD or HV-CD. With this above description, a diagnosis of iMCD-NOS is considered when a differentiation between HHV-8-associated Castleman disease and plasma cell Castleman disease cannot be made. Lastly, a mixed type of Castleman disease has been described in literature where both HV-CD and PC-CD co-exist in the same patient.

7. Clinical manifestations

Clinical manifestations of Castleman disease are varied and depend on the specific organ involved. However, generalizations regarding clinical symptoms can be drawn from various data available in literature, which are described below.

7.1 Unicentric Castleman disease

UCD is predominantly characterized by involvement of solitary nodal regions and typically demonstrates a benign course where progressive enlargement of the lesion ensues [32–34]. The median age is usually in the fourth decade, but it can involve patients of all age groups. Hyaline vascular Castleman disease (HV-CD) does not show any gender preponderance. Patients with HV-CD are often clinically asymptomatic, and a solitary lesion is incidentally detected during routine physical examination and / or imaging study.

HV-CD usually involves lymph nodes, especially supradiaphragmatic nodes (favor involvement of mediastinal lymph nodes or spleen, occasionally it can involve other extranodal sites. Occasionally, abdominal LNs can be involved, particularly in stromal-rich cases.

Symptoms that occur in HV-CD are usually secondary to mass effect due to the lymph nodal masses, which can include dyspnea on exertion, cough, or dysphagia. On rare occasion, HV-CD may present with paraneoplastic pemphigus in <5% of patients. An even rare association is myasthenia gravis in a patient with HV-CD.

Laboratory abnormalities and systemic symptoms are seldom seen in patients with HV variant of UCD, although a minor subset of patients may show elevated non-specific markers of inflammation like lactate dehydrogenase (LDH).

Plasma cell variant of Castleman disease (PC-CD) tends to occur at all ages but peaks during the fourth decade, and similar to HV-CD, there is no gender bias in PC-CD. It usually involves lymph nodes, but the relative involvement of the mediastinum is lesser in comparison with HV-CD. Patients are generally devoid of symptoms at presentation, and nodes/lesions are detected incidentally, but systemic symptoms and laboratory abnormalities have been reported in a small subset of patients.

In patients with PC-CD presenting with systemic symptoms, all efforts should be made to rule out multicentric Castleman disease as iMCD-NOS is a very important differential for the same. Most common symptoms that occur with PC-CD are B symptoms which often include fever, night sweats, weight loss, and malaise. Laboratory studies most commonly show blood abnormalities like anemia or a low platelet count. Owing to the dysregulation in IL-6 as the underlying pathology of PC-CD, lab testing for serum IL-6 levels shows raised levels in this subset of patients.

7.2 Multicentric Castleman disease

MCD occurs at varied age groups, with no specific gender predisposition. Symptoms related to multicentric Castleman disease are predominantly due to site of the lesions [35–37]. Multiple sites are usually involved with spleen in 75% of cases, and liver involvement seen in 50% of cases of MCD. Other clinical manifestations include Anasarca, Ascites, and skin rash among the most common symptoms. Similar to PC-CD, MCD patients may also present with B-symptoms in a similar manner to lymphoma which includes fever, night sweats, weight loss, and malaise, but about 90 to 95% of patients with MCD are found to present with B symptoms at the outset. The symptoms of multicentric CD are variable and may show a waxing-waning pattern.

Apart from clinical symptoms, lab abnormalities are very common in patients with MCD. Bone marrow abnormalities like anemia and thrombocytopenia, immune abnormalities in the form of polyclonal hypergammaglobulinemia, and non-specific markers of inflammation which include Elevated ESR, Elevated IL-6 levels, LDH, IFN-¥, and CRP are noted in patients with Castleman disease. Renal involvement is also commonly seen in patients with MCD (60% of patients).

8. Investigations and diagnosis

Castleman disease (CD) is typically a histological diagnosis, but the suspicion of CD is often based on imaging findings and an astute clinician. Various imaging modalities and laboratory tests can be done to evaluate a patient with CD which are depicted in **Figure 3** as per recommendations of the National Comprehensive Cancer Network v.1.2025, which

Diagnostic Workup in Castleman Disease

Essential:

1. Incisional/Excisional Biopsy
2. Adequate IHC Panel: CD20, CD3, HHV8, LANA
3. Physical Exam
4. Performance Status
5. Assessment for "Active Disease"
6. CBC with Differential
7. LDH, CRP, ESR
8. SPEP and Urine Electrophoresis
9. PET/CT (preferred) or CT T/A/P with contrast
10. Pregnancy testing in women of childbearing age
11. HIV, Hepatitis B, HHV8, EBV PCR
12. 2D Echocardiography

Optional:

1. Molecular analysis to detect Ig rearrangements
2. IHC Panel: Ki-67, Ig heavy chains, CD5,CD10, BCL2, BCL6, Cyclin D1
3. EBER-ISH (EBV-encoded RNA in situ hybridization)
4. Bone Marrow Biopsy + Aspirate
5. Reticulin fibrosis of bone marrow
6. Contrast CT of the neck
7. Multigated acquisition scan (plan of anthracycline based regimen)
8. IgG4, sIL6, sIL10, VEGF, Uric acid, Ferritin

Fertility Preservation to be discussed (in all men and women of reproductive age group

Figure 3.
Diagnostic workup in CD.

broadly include essential workup (these tests need to be done in all patients of CD) and optional (to be done if available, or in certain subtypes of CD). The modalities include laboratory studies, ultrasonography, CT, MRI, and/or PET-CT scan [32–34].

8.1 Laboratory studies

Lab studies are usually ancillary tests in patients with CD and do not provide a diagnostic confirmation [32]. As described earlier, patients with UCD usually have normal labs, whereas patients with MCD can have lab abnormalities based on the subtype. Histopathologic examination is often the confirmatory test for patients with CD. Excisional biopsy from the lymph node is generally considered as the gold standard for diagnosis owing to its greater tissue yield and the propensity to run additional immunohistochemical and molecular tests in a single sample. An optional investigation is an incisional biopsy which gives cores of tissue for analysis. Fine needle aspiration is usually nondiagnostic and is not currently recommended as per the NCCN guidelines.

8.2 Plain radiographs

Chest radiograph is often the first imaging modality in the evaluation of lung pathology [32, 33]. Patients with UCD involving the thorax may manifest as an incidental mediastinal mass with or without pleural effusion. In such a presentation, common differentials such a tuberculosis, lung cancer, and other benign and malignant tumors of the lung should be evaluated for prior to labelling a patient with CD. Radiographs are usually not useful in evaluating other organs such as abdominal viscera, and these require advanced modalities such as CT/MRI.

8.3 Computed tomography

Computed tomography (CT) is a widely and the most used tool to evaluate a patient with CD [34]. The CT features vary with the type of Castleman disease. The typical appearance of UCD is a described as a solitary, well-circumscribed, enlarged lymph node, or localized nodal mass. On non-contrast CT images, the nodes are hypodense in comparison with skeletal muscle, with homogeneous contrast enhancement which signifies hypervascularity of the lesion. The lesions are most commonly seen to affect the thorax and abdominal regions. In addition, CT can also guide in the biopsy of the lesions for a histopathological diagnosis.

MCD typically manifests as multiple generalized lymphadenopathy usually involving bilateral hilar and/or mediastinal lymphadenopathy. Abdominal lesions are common in patients with MCD where a well-defined enhancing lesion may be noted in the abdomen, in addition to retroperitoneal, mesenteric, or porta hepatis disease or diffuse abdominal lymphadenopathy. Other intra-thoracic manifestations include involvement of the lung parenchyma (with a cystic lung disease pattern which mimics a lymphocytic interstitial pneumonia pattern). Alternatively, enhancing pulmonary masses, pleural effusion, septal thickening, and consolidations may also be noted in patients with MCD. Other systemic manifestations such as hepatosplenomegaly / ascites may be seen.

8.4 MRI

MRI is also useful in the evaluation of CD as it not only shows the extent of the lesions, but it can also show relationships to the adjacent structures, especially vessels and soft tissues [34]. Most CD lesions are either isointense or slightly hyperintense relative to skeletal muscle on T1-weighted images and hyperintense on T2-weighted images, which reflects the vascularity of the masses. MRI can also demonstrate the feeding vessels as flow void structures. Central linear hypointense septate may be seen and has been suggested to represent reticulin fibrosis.

8.5 Ultrasonography

Ultrasonography is a ubiquitous, simple, and inexpensive tool available for the evaluation of peripheral, abdominal, and/or pelvic lesions [34]. Most lesions in patients with Castleman disease appear as nonspecific, well-defined hypoechoic masses without necrosis on ultrasonography. Other findings which favor a diagnosis of Castleman disease are the presence of prominent peripheral vessels around the mass, with feeding vessels demonstrated on Doppler study. Post-acoustic shadowing of involved lesions has also been described in patients with Castleman disease. Similar appearances maybe seen in lymphoma, sarcoidosis, and tuberculosis especially in the early stage (before conglomeration has occurred).

8.6 PET

Positron emission tomography (PET-CT) is part of nuclear imaging, and it gives information regarding the metabolic activity of a lymph node/nodal masses in a patient with CD [34]. It also adds to the prognosis in patients with CD on treatment to assess response to therapy. Fluorodeoxyglucose F 18 (18F-FDG) avid lesions has been demonstrated in patients with active Castleman disease. Increased 18F-FDG uptake is suggestive of an active lesion, and a PET-non avid lesion goes in favor of an inactive lesion. The SUV values of patients with UCD and MCD are in general lesser in comparison with SUV uptake in other diseases such as malignancy or lymphomas. PET may also aid in localizing asymptomatic or small lesions, which may otherwise not be picked up using ancillary imaging techniques. In addition, 18F-FDG–PET/CT can also aid in sampling of the lesion (a PET avid lesion is likely to yield a better diagnosis in comparison with a PET non-avid lesion).

Overall, diagnosis of Castleman disease takes a multifaceted approach, where neither one test can replace the other, and they complement each other in confirmation of the diagnosis.

The standard workflow in the diagnosis of a patient with CD is given in **Figure 4**, and the consensus diagnostic criteria are given in **Table 2**. (put forth by NCCN, Fagjenbaum et al., and van Rhee et al.). Additionally, criteria for active disease is put forth in **Figure 5**.

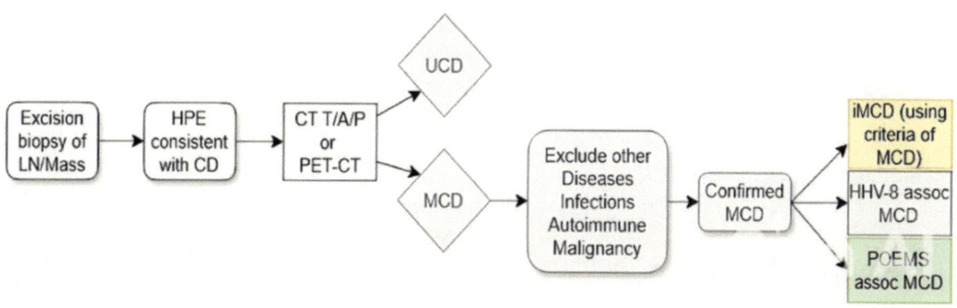

Figure 4.
Diagnostic pathway for a patient with suspected Castleman disease.

Consensus criteria for Castleman disease (Taken from NCCN Guidelines [38], also concurs with Fajgenbaum et al. [39]; and van Rhee et al. [40]) [38–40]
1. The presence of both major criteria • Histopathologic lymph node features consistent with the iMCD spectrum. Features along the iMCD spectrum include (need grade 2–3 for either regressive GCs or plasmacytosis at minimum): i. Regressed/atrophic/atretic germinal centers, often with expanded mantle zones composed of concentric rings of lymphocytes in an "onion skinning" appearance – ii. FDC prominence iii. Vascularity, often with prominent endothelium in the interfollicular space and vessels penetrating the GCs with a "lollipop" appearance iv. Sheetlike, polytypic plasmacytosis in the interfollicular space—hyperplastic GCs
2. Enlarged lymph nodes ($\geq$1 cm in short-axis diameter) in $\geq$2 lymph node stations
3. The presence of at least 2/11 minor criteria (including at least 1 laboratory criterion)
Clinical symptoms 1. B symptoms (night sweats, fever over 38°, weight loss, or fatigue) 2. Splenomegaly and/or hepatomegaly 3. Edema, anasarca, ascites, pleural effusions 4. Lymphocytoid interstitial pneumonia 5. "Eruptive" hemangiomatoses
Laboratory criteria 1. Elevated C-reactive protein (>10 mg/L) or blood sedimentation (>15 mm/h) 2. Anemia (hemoglobin <12.5 g/dL men, <11.5 g/dL women) 3. Thrombocytopenia (<150/μL) or thrombocytosis (>400/μL) 4. Hypoalbuminemia (<3.5 g/dL) 5. Renal function impairment (eGFR <60 mL/min/1.73 m2) or proteinuria (total protein 150 mg/24 h or 10 mg/100 mL) 6. Polyclonal hypergammaglobulinemia (>1700 mg/dL)
4. Exclusion of other diseases with "Castleman-like" histology • Infection-associated diseases i. HHV-8 (PCR, serology, and/or LANA staining in the lymph node) ii. Infectious mononucleosis (EBV otherwise no exclusion criterion) iii. Lymphadenopathy (due to HIV, CMV, toxoplasmosis, tuberculosis) • Defined autoimmune diseases (detected antibodies alone do not exclude iMCD) such as systemic lupus erythematosus, rheumatoid arthritis, adult-onset Still's disease, juvenile idiopathic arthritis, and autoimmune lymphoproliferative syndrome • Malignant or lymphoproliferative diseases, diagnosed at the same time (Hodgkin's and non-Hodgkin's lymphomas, multiple myeloma, plasmacytoma localized primarily in the lymph node, and FDC sarcoma).

Table 2.
Diagnostic criteria for Castleman disease.

9. Differential diagnoses

Castleman disease has a wide range of differentials owing to the number of diseases that can present with mediastinal and abdominal lymphadenopathy.

Criteria for Active Disease

1.Fever
2.Increased serum C-reactive protein level >20 mg/L in the absence of any other etiology
3.At least three of the following other MCD-related symptoms:
·Peripheral lymphadenopathy
·Enlarged spleen
·Edema
·Pleural effusion
·Ascites
·Cough
·Nasal obstruction
·Xerostomia
·Rash
·CNS symptoms
·Jaundice
·Autoimmune hemolytic anemia

Figure 5.
Criteria for active disease in CD.

The list of differentials is given below

1. Autoimmune diseases

    a. Rheumatoid arthritis

    b. Systemic lupus erythematosus

    c. Still' disease (adult onset)

    d. Juvenile rheumatoid arthritis

2. Infectious diseases

    a. Ebstein–Barr virus

    b. CMV

    c. Tuberculosis

    d. HIV

    e. Toxoplasmosis

3. Malignancies

    a. Hodgkin's lymphoma

    b. Non-Hodgkin's lymphoma

    c. Lung carcinoma

4. Miscellaneous diseases

    a. IgG4 disease

10. Diagnostic criteria for Castleman disease

See **Table 2**.

11. Management

As already discussed, due to the varying histopathology, etiopathogenesis, and the relative rarity of the diagnosis of Castleman disease, consensus classification for diagnosis and management was introduced as late as 2017 and 2018 [15, 41].

Needless to say, a systematic approach and a high index of suspicion is required for the management of patients with Castleman disease, and the main confounder for this is its relative rarity and heterogeneity.

Furthermore, patients with associated conditions, such as infection with HIV/HHV-8 or other comorbidities, may require special consideration.

The latest article from the National Comprehensive Cancer Network (NCCN) guideline for management of CD is currently available [42].

The algorithmic management of unicentric Castleman disease is given in **Figure 6**. For patients with unicentric Castleman disease, upfront surgery or radiation to localized area is the management of choice. With surgical removal being almost always successful for unicentric disease, irrespective of the variant. Unicentric CD has a good prognosis with a 95% response rate. Dr. Benjamin Castleman was the initial proposer that surgery is a definite curative modality of management for Castleman disease.

If the disease is unresectable, then first-line chemotherapeutic agents should be used. Additional options include chemoembolization of the lesion by interventional radiology.

Unlike UCD, iMCD is a systemic disease with potentially life-threatening possibility.

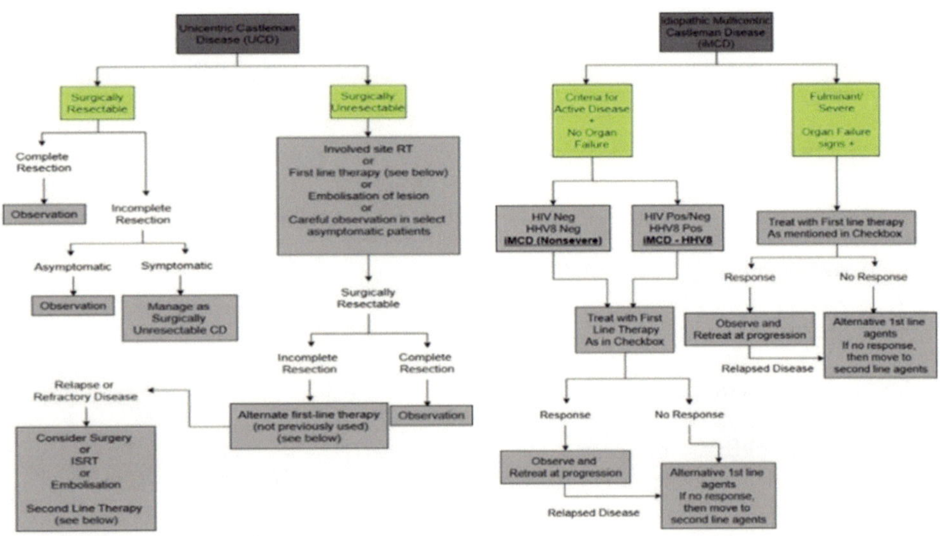

Figure 6.
Algorithm for management of Castleman disease.

First Line Therapy Options

UCD:

- ·Rituximab
- ·Rituximab + cyclophosphamide
- ·Rituximab + prednisone
- ·Rituximab + prednisone + cyclophosphamide

MCD:

- ·HHV8-negative/HIV-1-negative (iMCD -Nonsevere)
- ·Rituximab
- ·Rituximab + prednisone
- ·RCVP (rituximab, cyclophosphamide, vincristine, prednisone)
- ·Siltuximab
- ·Thalidomide + cyclophosphamide + prednisone
- HHV8-positive (HIV-1-positive or HIV-1-negative)
- ·Rituximab (preferred)
- ·Rituximab + liposomal doxorubicin Rituximab + prednisone
- ·Rituximab + prednisone + liposomal doxorubicin
- ·Zidovudine + ganciclovir/valganciclovir

MCD – Fulminant/ Organ Failure

Fulminant/severe HHV8-negative (iMCD)

- CHOP (cyclophosphamide, doxorubicin, vincristine, prednisone) ± rituximab
- CVAD (cyclophosphamide, vincristine, doxorubicin, and dexamethasone) ± rituximab
- CVP (cyclophosphamide, vincristine, prednisone) ± rituximab
- Siltuximab
- If not a candidate for combination therapy: Rituximab

Fulminant/severe HHV8-positive MCD

- Rituximab + liposomal doxorubicin
- Rituximab + prednisone + liposomal doxorubicin
- RCHOP (rituximab, cyclophosphamide, doxorubicin, vincristine, prednisone)
- RCVAD (rituximab, cyclophosphamide, vincristine, doxorubicin, and dexamethasone)
- RCVP (rituximab, cyclophosphamide, vincristine, and prednisone)
- If not a candidate for combination therapy:
- Liposomal doxorubicin
- Rituximab

Figure 7.
Treatment of unicentric and multicentric Castleman disease.

Second Line Agents (For Relapse/ Progressive / Refractory Disease)

·Anakinra
·Bortezomib ± rituximab
·Lenalidomide ± rituximab
·Thalidomide ± rituximab
·Tocilizumab
·High-dose zidovudine + valganciclovir (if HHV8-positive)
·Sirolimus
·Vinblastine
·Siltuximab or tocilizumab (if HIV1-negative/HHV8-negative)

Figure 8.
Second line agents used in CD.

Surgical intervention is not the upfront standard of care in a patient with iMCD. iMCD treatment options include chemotherapy, and the recommended regimen and algorithm for management are given in **Figures 6**, **7**, and **8**, respectively.

As previously discussed in the pathogenesis section, the pivotal cytokine responsible for development of CD appears to be Interleukin-6(IL-6), and blockade of the IL-6 pathway using IL-6 receptor antagonists or monoclonal antibodies leads to elimination of the cells responsible for cytokine overproduction. Other agents which have been used and studied in iMCD include rituximab which has been used with and without cytotoxic agents. Immunomodulatory therapies, especially steroids, have also been used in the management of Castleman disease.

Even with the prescribed regimens, about 50% patients fail to respond to the first line recommended treatment options of siltuximab, tocilizumab, or rituximab. A monoclonal antibody that was approved for iMCD in 2013 was siltuximab, and due to clinical trials which showed a favorable response to siltuximab vs. placebo [38], it has currently been recommended as the first-line agent for all forms of iMCD. In the landmark trial of siltuximab vs. placebo, there was a 34% greater response in siltuximab vs. placebo.

Other drugs recommended for relapse/refractory disease include Tocilizumab, Sirolimus - mTOR inhibitor, Vinblastine, Thalidomide, and Anakinra.

12. Prognosis and follow-up

Castleman disease is a heterogeneous disorder, and its pathogenesis is very complex and multifactorial [8, 39, 40, 43, 44]. Hence, standard treatments established for CD are based on few randomized trials and case series and expert consensus statements [15, 41, 42]. Additionally, only a handful of research material is available on the prognostic factors of CD [39–41, 43, 44], especially in HHV-8 negative patients. Regarding CD, there are significant differences with respect to treatment and prognosis among patients with UCD and MCD.

In cases of unicentric CD, complete resection of the involved lesion is considered as the standard of care and is often considered curative (it was also the first therapy suggested by Castleman et al. in the year 1954), [1, 2], and the 5-year OS rate is about 95–100%.

Unlike UCD, the prognosis of iMCD is poor and more prone to relapses and progression. A variety of chemotherapeutic agents have been used to treat iMCD according to the histological variant, and based on disease severity (fulminant or organ threatening disease), which includes but is not limited to corticosteroids, chemotherapeutic agents, thalidomide, immunoglobulin, rituximab, anti-IL-6 antibody (siltuximab and tocilizumab), and mTOR pathway inhibitors. Detailed regimens are given in checkboxes in the management section.

Among the various studies reviewed [39–41, 43, 44] regarding prognosis and the factors which contributed to poor or worse prognosis in CD patients, most studies concurred with the following factors

- Hemoglobin <10 g/dl
- Albumin <3 g/dl
- Serous effusion
- Hepatosplenomegaly
- Leukopenia (TLC <4000 cells/mm^{3})
- Age > 60 years
- Presence of B symptoms
- Performance status.

A multivariate analysis conducted in a study by Liu et al. [39] showed that PC subtype, hepatomegaly and/or splenomegaly, hemoglobin ≤80 g/L, and albumin ≤30 g/L were independent contributors to poor prognosis among iMCD patients. A CECT T/A/P or a PET-CT should be used for ascertaining response which is characterized into complete response, partial response, and no response. ESR, CRP, and LDH levels also can be used for prognosticating CD patients, but more studies are required to ascertain standardized cut-off values. A prognostic scoring which was assessed in iMCD is given in the **Table 3** [44].

Characteristic	Level of severity		
	Mild	Intermediate	Severe
ECOG PS	0–1	—	≥2
Renal function	Normal	—	CrCl <30 ml/min
Fluid overload	Absent	—	Anasarca/Ascites
Hb	≥10		≤8
Pulmonary involvement	Absent	—	Present

Table 3.
Prognostic factors in Castleman disease.

Conflict of interest

The author declares no conflict of interest.

Acronyms and abbreviations

CD:	Castleman disease
AIDS	acquired immunodeficiency syndrome
CD-XX	cluster of differentiation-XX
CMV	cytomegalovirus
CRP	c-reactive protein
CT	computed tomography
CXCL13	chemokine ligand 13
EBV	ebstein–barr virus
ECOG	eastern cooperative oncology group
ESR	erythrocyte sedimentation rate
Hb	hemoglobin
HHV-8	human herpesvirus-8
HIV	human immunodeficiency virus
HV-CD	hyaline vascular variant of Castleman disease
ICD	international classification of diseases.
IGg4	immunoglobulin g4
IL-1B	interleukin 1 beta
IL-6	interleukin 6
iMCD	idiopathic multicentric Castleman disease
iMCD-NOS	idiopathic multicentric Castleman disease—Not otherwise specified
JAK/STAT	Janus kinase/signal transducer and activator of transcription
JNK	c-Jun N-terminal kinase
KSHV	kaposi sarcoma herpesvirus
LDH	lactate dehydrogenase
MAPK	Ras-mitogen-activated protein kinase
MCD	multicentric Castleman disease
MRI	magnetic resonance imaging
NCCN	national comprehensive cancer network
PC-CD	plasma cell variant of Castleman disease
PCs	plasma cells

PET-CT	positron emission tomography
PI3K/mTOR	phosphoinositide 3-kinase/mammalian target of rapamycin
POEMS	polyneuropathy, organomegaly, endocrinopathy, M protein, and skin changes
PS	performance status
TAFRO	thrombocytopenia, anasarca, fever/elevated C-reactive protein (CRP), renal dysfunction/reticulin myelofibrosis, organomegaly
TLC	total leukocyte count
UCD	unicentric Castleman disease
VEGF	vascular endothelial growth factor

Author details

Prakash Sivaramakrishnan
National Institute of Tuberculosis and Respiratory Diseases, New Delhi, India

*Address all correspondence to: sprakash1989@gmail.com

References

[1] Castleman B, Towne VW. CASE records of the Massachusetts general hospital weekly clinicopathological exercises: CASE 40011. The New England Journal of Medicine. 1954;**250**:26-30

[2] Castleman B, Iverson L, Menendez VP. Localized mediastinal lymph-node hyperplasia resembling thymoma. Cancer. 1956;**9**:822-830

[3] Flendrig JA. Benign giant lymphoma: Clinicopathologic correlation study. In: Clark RL, Gumley RW, editors. The Year Book of Cancer. Chicago: Year Book Medical Publishers; 1970. pp. 296-299

[4] Keller AR, Hochholzer L, Castleman B. Hyaline-vascular and plasma-cell types of giant lymph node hyperplasia of the mediastinum and other locations. Cancer. 1972;**29**:670-683

[5] Chang Y, Cesarman E, Pessin MS, et al. Identification of herpesvirus-like DNA sequences in AIDS-associated Kaposi's sarcoma. Science. 1994;**266**(5192):1865-1869

[6] Simpson D. Epidemiology of Castleman disease. Hematology/Oncology Clinics of North America. 2018;**32**(1):1-10

[7] Munshi N, Mehra M, van de Velde H, et al. Use of a claims database to characterize and estimate the incidence rate for Castleman disease. Leukemia & Lymphoma. 2015;**56**(5):1252-1260

[8] Katherine, Heyland DRJ, Daniel T, Grima TS, et al. Preliminary prevalence estimate of multicentric Castleman's disease in Asia-Pacific. ISH. 2014:14-23

[9] Chen KT. Multicentric Castleman's disease and Kaposi's sarcoma. The American Journal of Surgical Pathology. 1984;**8**:287-293

[10] Iwaki N, Fajgenbaum DC, Nabel CS, et al. Clinicopathologic analysis of TAFRO syndrome demonstrates a distinct subtype of HHV-8-negative multicentric Castleman disease. American Journal of Hematology. 2016;**91**(2):220-226

[11] Bardwick PA, Zvaifler NJ, Gill GN, et al. Plasma cell dyscrasia with polyneuropathy, organomegaly, endocrinopathy, M protein, and skin changes: The POEMS syndrome. Report on two cases and a review of the literature. Medicine. 1980;**59**(4):311-322

[12] Masaki Y, Kawabata H, Takai K, et al. Proposed diagnostic criteria, disease severity classification and treatment strategy for TAFRO syndrome, 2015 version. International Journal of Hematology. 2016;**103**(6):686-692

[13] Yoshizaki K, Murayama S, Ito H, Koga T. The role of interleukin-6 in Castleman disease. Hematology/Oncology Clinics of North America. 2018;**32**(1):23-36. DOI: 10.1016/j.hoc.2017.09.003

[14] Wang W, Liu Z, Zhao X. Overview of research status in Castleman disease. Clinical Lymphoma Myeloma and Leukemia. 2024;**24**(10):e359-e365

[15] Fajgenbaum DC, Uldrick TS, Bagg A, et al. International, evidence-based consensus diagnostic criteria for HHV-8-negative/idiopathic multicentric Castleman disease. Blood. 2017;**129**(12):1646-1657. DOI: 10.1182/blood-2016-10-746933

[16] Wing A, Xu J, Meng W, et al. Transcriptome and unique cytokine

microenvironment of Castleman disease. Modern Pathology. 2022;**35**(4):451-461. DOI: 10.1038/ s41379- 021- 00950- 3

[17] Brito MT, Amador AF, Moço Coutinho R, Ribeiro A, Almeida JS. Human herpesvirus-8 (HHV-8)-positive human immunodeficiency virus (HIV) negative multicentric castleman disease with a fulminant course. Cureus. 2024;**16**(2):e54350. DOI: 10.7759/ cureus.54350

[18] Sekiguchi Y, Misawa S, Shibuya K, et al. Ambiguous effects of anti-VEGF monoclonal antibody (bevacizumab) for POEMS syndrome. Journal of Neurology, Neurosurgery, and Psychiatry. 2013;**84**(12):1346-1348

[19] Pierson SK, Stonestrom AJ, Shilling D, et al. Plasma proteomics identifies a 'chemokine storm' in idiopathic multicentric Castleman disease. American Journal of Hematology. 2018;**93**(7):902-912. DOI: 10.1002/ajh.25123

[20] You L, Lin Q, Zhao J, Shi F, Young KH, Qian W. Whole-exome sequencing identifies novel somatic alterations associated with outcomes in idiopathic multicentric Castleman disease. British Journal of Haematology. 2020;**188**(5):e64-e67. DOI: 10.1111/ bjh.16330

[21] Fajgenbaum DC, Shilling D. Castleman disease pathogenesis. Hematology/Oncology Clinics of North America. 2018;**32**(1):11-21

[22] Aguzzi A, Kranich J, Krautler NJ. Follicular dendritic cells: Origin, phenotype, and function in health and disease. Trends in Immunology. 2014;**35**(3):105-113

[23] Guihot A, Oksenhendler E, Galicier L, et al. Multicentric Castleman disease is associated with polyfunctional effector memory HHV-8-specific CD8 T cells. Blood. 2008;**111**(3):1387-1395

[24] Uldrick TS, Polizzotto MN, Yarchoan R. Recent advances in Kaposi sarcoma herpesvirus-associated multicentric Castleman disease. Current Opinion in Oncology. 2012;**24**(5):495-505

[25] Wu D, Lim MS, Jaffe ES. Pathology of Castleman disease. Hematology/ Oncology Clinics of North America. 2018;**32**(1):37-52

[26] Yu L, Tu M, Cortes J, et al. Clinical and pathological characteristics of HIV- and HHV-8-negative Castleman disease. Blood. 2017;**129**(12):1658-1668

[27] Frizzera G, Banks PM, Massarelli G, et al. A systemic lymphoproliferative disorder with morphologic features of Castleman's disease. Pathological findings in 15 patients. The American Journal of Surgical Pathology. 1983;**7**(3):211-231

[28] Wang W, Medeiros LJ. Castleman disease. Surgical Pathology Clinics. 2019;**12**(3):849-863

[29] Ruco LP, Gearing AJ, Pigott R, et al. Expression of ICAM-1, VCAM-1 and ELAM-1 in angiofollicular lymph node hyperplasia (Castleman's disease): Evidence for dysplasia of follicular dendritic reticulum cells. Histopathology. 1991;**19**:523-528

[30] Chang KC, Wang YC, Hung LY, et al. Monoclonality and cytogenetic abnormalities in hyaline vascular Castleman disease. Modern Pathology. 2014;**27**:823-831

[31] Cronin DM, Warnke RA. Castleman disease: An update on classification and the spectrum of associated lesions.

Advances in Anatomic Pathology. 2009;**16**(4):236-246

[32] Hoffmann C, Oksenhendler E, Littler S, Grant L, Kanhai K, Fajgenbaum DC. The clinical picture of Castleman disease: A systematic review and meta-analysis. Blood Advances. 2024;**8**(18):4924-4935

[33] Carbone A, Borok M, Damania B, Gloghini A, Polizzotto MN, Jayanthan RK, et al. Castleman disease. Nature Reviews. Disease Primers. 2021;**7**(1):84

[34] Bonekamp D, Horton KM, Hruban RH, Fishman EK. Castleman disease: The great mimic. Radiographics. 2011;**31**(6):1793-1807

[35] Zhou T, Wang HW, Pittaluga S, Jaffe ES. Multicentric Castleman disease and the evolution of the concept. Pathologica. 2021;**113**(5):339-353

[36] Masaki Y, Arita K, Sakai T, Takai K, Aoki S, Kawabata H. Castleman disease and TAFRO syndrome. Annals of Hematology. 2022;**101**(3):485-490

[37] Piris MA, Aguirregoicoa E, Montes-Moreno S, Celeiro-Muñoz C. Castleman disease and Rosai-Dorfman disease. Seminars in Diagnostic Pathology. 2018;**35**(1):44-53

[38] van Rhee F, Wong RS, Munshi N, Rossi JF, Ke XY, Fosså A, et al. Siltuximab for multicentric Castleman's disease: A randomised, double-blind, placebo-controlled trial. The Lancet Oncology. 2014;**15**(9):966-974. DOI: 10.1016/S1470-2045(14)70319-5

[39] Liu W, Cai Q, Yu T, Strati P, Hagemeister FB, Zhai Q et al. Clinical characteristics and outcomes of Castleman disease: A multicenter consortium study of 428 patients with 15-year follow-up. American Journal of Cancer Research. 15 Sep 2022;**12**(9):4227-4240

[40] Zhang X, Rao H, Xu X, Li Z, Liao B, Wu H, et al. Clinical characteristics and outcomes of Castleman disease: A multicenter study of 185 Chinese patients. Cancer Science. 2018;**109**(1):199-206

[41] Lang E, Van Rhee F. Idiopathic multicentric Castleman disease: An update in diagnosis and treatment advances. Blood Reviews. 2024;**64**:101161

[42] NCCN Clinical Practice Guidelines in Oncology (NCCN Guidelines®) Castleman Disease Version 1.2025. 2024 [Accessed: December 28, 2024]

[43] Zhang L, Li Z, Cao X, Feng J, Zhong D, Wang S, et al. Clinical spectrum and survival analysis of 145 cases of HIV-negative Castleman's disease: Renal function is an important prognostic factor. Scientific Reports. 2016;**6**(1):23831

[44] Min GJ, Jeon YW, Kim TY, Kwag DH, Lee JH, Lee JY, et al. Long-term treatment outcome of Castleman's disease: A real-world experience. Frontiers in Oncology. 2022;**12**:974770

Chapter 7

The Classifications of the Lower Limb Lymphedemas by the Belgian Society of Lymphology Based on Clinical and Lympho-Scintigraphic Data

Pierre Bourgeois, Mirela Mariana Roman, Romain Barbieux, Joseph Harfouche and Olivier Leduc

Abstract

The reading of articles on limb lymphedema often appears imprecise, particularly when focusing on the associated lympho-scintigraphic images that describe and define them. Their definitions, analyses, and reports need to be standardized. In the present chapter, the members of the Belgian Society of Lymphology propose and develop an approach that leads to a rational classification of these lymphedemas, and present their definitions and proposals for standardizing these different images and their reporting. In this chapter, only the issue of lower limb edema will be addressed.

Keywords: lymphatic imaging, lympho-scintigraphy, lower limb lymphedema, definitions, classification, BeSL, BeSL severity score index-classification for lymphatic Edemas

1. Introduction

Lymphedema affects a significant number of patients worldwide. Beyond the well-studied secondary upper limb lymphedema post-breast cancer treatment, the lower limb forms (LLLE) remain insufficiently standardized, particularly regarding their classification. The literature concerning these edemas reveals very heterogeneous populations and equally diverse situations, often grouped under the somewhat simplified and "generalist" term "lymphedema" [1]. Additionally, although lymphoscintigraphic examinations (LySc) are considered the gold standard reference [2], their methodologies appear very variable, and the reading of articles on lower limb lymphedema often seems imprecise when focusing on the associated lympho-scintigraphic images that define them [3–13].

The Belgian Society of Lymphology (BeSL), whose members are all directly or indirectly involved in the management of these edemas and are familiar in the use of different imaging techniques of the lymphatic system, including lymphoscintigraphies, proposes a new approach to classifying lower limb lymphedemas based on both clinical and lympho-scintigraphic findings. This approach is inspired by the TNM cancer classification system and seeks to offer a structured and reproducible framework for diagnosis, phenotyping, therapeutic guidance, and evaluation.

2. From one "disease" to several clinical entities: One "lymphedema"? Multiple lymphedemas! The approach for the classification of the lymphedemas by the Belgian Society of Lymphology (BeSL)

If cancer is a disease that can affect all organs of the human body, these cancers are all different, and cancers affecting a specific organ can show the characteristics that practically make them subgroups requiring adapted management [14]. It is therefore proposed to classify these lymphedemas into groups based on their basic clinical characteristics (see **Table 1**).

2.1.1 Group 1: the "syndromic" lymphedemas (S-LE) when associated with a "multi-organ" disease.
2.1.2 Group 2: the "primary" lymphedema (1ary-LE) are said "congenital" (when present at birth), "sporadic" by opposition to the following, and "familial" cases where multiple family members have lymph-edema (and a genetic anomaly should be investigated). These primary lymphedemas are also called "early-onset" (or "praecox) when diagnosed before the age of 35 years and "late-onset" (or "tarda") after this age.
2.1.3 Group 3: the "secondary" lymphedemas (2ary-LE)
2.1.3.1 Secondary to cancer, the "cancer-related-lymphedema" (CR-LE).
We distinguish different groups here:

- Secondary to extensive lymph node dissection alone (CRL-LNx)
- Secondary to a sentinel procedure, to a selective lymphadenectomy alone (CRL-LNs)
- Secondary to radiotherapy alone (CRL-Rxt)
- Secondary to chemotherapy alone (CRL-Cht)
- Secondary to a treatment combining different therapeutic interventions (CRL LN+/−Rxt+/-Cht)
- Secondary in the context of a newly discovered cancer with multiple lymph node involvement (CRL-LNm)
- Secondary in the context of progressive cancer with multiple lymph node involvement (CRL LNe)

2.1.3.2 Phlebo-lymphedemas, edemas of the lower limbs associated with venous abnormalities (P-LE)
2.1.3.3 Edemas related to nervous pathology, like hemiplegia (N-LE)
2.1.3.4 Edemas in the context of an infectious disease (like filariosis) affecting the lymphatic system (I-LE)
2.1.3.5 Edemas associated with osteoarticular pathology (arthritis, fracture, complex regional pain syndrome, etc.) (BA-LE)
2.1.3.6 Edemas associated with a systemic disease (like Fabry disease) (SL)
2.1.4 Group 4: the "lipedemas" (Ap-LE). Lipedemas represent a particular group where the disease actually concerns adipose tissue [15, 16], and where anomalies of the lymphatic system are observed and considered secondary in the context of this disease.
2.1.5 Group 5: the "Not-Otherwise-Classified" (NOC) lymphedema: For example, the diagnosis of lymphedema in a morbidly obese patient without any identifiable genetic or oncologic cause but with clear lymphoscintigraphic evidence of impaired drainage [17] may fall under the NOC category. Similarly, post-infectious limb swelling following erysipelas with no further recurrence but persistent edema and patients with "paradoxical lymphedema" (where the lympho-scintigraphic investigations of the superficial lymphatic system show one functional response of the edematous limb either as good as or better than the one of the normal limb) [18] would also belong to this group. Such edematous situations need additional investigations, of the venous return, of the deep lymphatic system, in searching osteo-articular disease, ... before being definitively "classified."

Table 1.
The BeSL "clinical" classification of the lower limb lymph-edemas (LLLE).

2.1 The BeSL VLM (TNM like) classifications of the lower limb lymph-edemas

By analogy with the TNM classification for cancers [14], where T is based on the size of the Tumor, N corresponds to the regional spread of the cancerous disease to the lymph nodes, and M to the presence of the disease in distant organ tissues, we are developing an equivalent that includes the different factors that seem to influence our therapeutic management of lower limb lymphedema and our understanding of their progression.

2.1.1 From T-nm to V-lm

The notion of T in cancers, if applied to lower limb edema, immediately raises various clinical issues, the location and extent of the edema, the issue of temporality (considering the history and previous progression of the edema at the time of its management, the issue of lower limb edemas extending to almost the entire limb), and the expression of these volumes.

It is necessary to distinguish between different types of distribution of these volume excesses, namely:

- "Distal" edema (Vd) only affecting the distal part of the limb (foot-ankle-calf)
- "Proximal" edema (Vp) only affecting the root of the limb (groin, upper thigh, possibly the pelvis and genital area)
- Isolated "segmental" edema (Vs-1) only affecting one segment of the lower limb between the foot and the groin but not extending to these two areas: For example, an edema limited to the ankle will be localized.
- "multi-segmental" edema (Vs-m x-y) initially affecting one or more segments of the lower limb but extending to the foot or the groin: or example, an edema limited to the ankle and distal part of the calf will be localized as Vs-m 2-3a.
- "Global" edema (Vw) affecting the entire limb from the foot to its root.

In most publications, the issue of edema volume is considered only globally and for the entire limb using circumferential measurements [19], often in comparison with the opposite limb, which is assumed to be normal. This approach seems us only valid and usable for unilateral edemas. Additionally, it neglects the clinical fact that some edemas may, for example, affect only the foot and/or ankle, sometimes the calf, the thigh alone, or the pelvis and genitals. Significant edema limited to the foot and ankle may be below the critical value set for the whole limb [19] but constitutes a major issue for the patients that cannot be under-estimated. Rather than defining edemas based on considering the entire limb, we prefer to define volume excesses in relation to the edematous areas themselves (either "in absolute terms" and in milliliters, or "relatively" and in percentages compared to the opposite territory).

2.1.2 From t-N-m to v-L-m or about lymphangio- and/or lymphadeno-, hypo-, and/or A-plasia

The terms hypoplasia, hyperplasia, dysplasia, and aplasia of the lymphatic system appear in the lymphatic medical literature as a continuation and development of the usage initially proposed by radiologists [20–23] based on their radiological images of these pathologies. Their description is mainly morphological.

When primary LLLE are suspected, we will use specifically the term "aplasia" to describe the lymphatic structures after interdigital injection seen on LySc [24]:

- only deep lymphatic vessels (dLV) are seen at the level of the calf with intercalated lymph nodes, sometimes without inferior inguinal LN = superficial Lymph-Vessel-aplasia or sLVA,

- inguinal and/or iliac LN are not seen or hypoactive = "Lympho-Nodal-Aplasia" (or LNA)

When injection is performed [18] in the retro-malleolar anterior space of the triceps surae tendon (Kager's triangle) to investigate the deep lymphatic drainage of the limb, we will also use specifically the term "aplasia" when no deep lymph vessels are seen running deep in the calf: sometimes with increased lymph flow at the level of the superficial LV of the edematous limb when compared to the normal limb = deep lympho-nodal aplasia or dLNA.

The term "hypoplasia" will be used to describe less clear situations after interdigital:

- both deep and superficial LV are observed with popliteal and/or sural intercalated LN = "superficial and/or deep lymph-vessel-hypoplasia" or sLVH-dLVH,

- inguinal and/or iliac LN are not seen or hypoactive = "lympho-nodal-hypoplasia" (or LNH)

- the tracer does not reach the inferior inguinal LN after 30 minutes phase 1 and/or after phase 2 and/or extraction is decreased under the value of 30% and/or extractions, nodal accumulations of the tracer after phases 1 and/or 2 show significant asymmetry = "lymph-system-hypoplasia" or LSH,

- inguinal and iliac LN are well seen but pLVR are seen = "proximal lympho-nodal-hypoplasia" (or pLNH).

2.1.3 From tn-M to vl-M with M is here "the changes of the oede-M-atous tissues"

It seems evident to us that we cannot consider recent-onset edemas and those that have evolved over years in the same way. The former can be limited, resolvable with simple maneuvers, present pitting (and be only fluid-related), and may not have skin or infectious complications. The latter are more often extensive, non-resolvable, no longer present pitting, may have been sites of infectious-inflammatory episodes, and show skin and underlying tissue changes (fibrosis and/or adipose tissue development).

The chronicity of lower limb edemas is thus expressed in the classification proposed by the ISL for these lower limb lymphedemas [1]. This staging of the ISL (which applies to the entire limb) mix clinical notions (the presence or absence of pitting, reduction of edema with limb elevation) and tissue changes that are subject to the subjectivity of the clinician and/or the patient.

Type 0: Clinical symptoms and/or para-clinical examinations results suggestive of edema of lymphatic origin. Pitting is absent. Latent lymphedema (with impaired lymph transport demonstrable with lymphoscintigraphy and with initial immunohistochemical alterations of lymph nodes, lymph vessels, and the extracellular matrix). They represent most frequently the "not-otherwise-classified" lymph-edemas.
Type 1 distal: Initial lymphedema at the level of the toes, foot, and/or ankle and/o distal part of the calf, with pitting positive (and Stemmer's sign sometimes positive), totally or partially relieved with rest, and a draining position (with worsening impairment of lymph drainage capacity and of the immunohistochemical alterations of lymph nodes, lymph vessels, and the extracellular matrix).
Type 1 segmental: Where edema is observed at the level of the ankle and/or calf with pitting positive, totally or partially relieved with rest and a draining position, (with worsening impairment of lymph drainage capacity and of the immunohistochemical alterations of lymph nodes, lymph vessels, and the extracellular matrix).
Type 2 distal: Initial lymphedema at the level of the toes, foot and/or ankle, and/o distal part of the calf, with pitting positive (and Stemmer's sign sometimes positive), NOT RELEIVING with rest and a draining position (with worsening impairment of lymph drainage capacity and of the immunohistochemical alterations of lymph nodes, lymph vessels, and the extracellular matrix).
Type 2 segmental: Where edema is observed at the level of the ankle and/or calf with pitting positive, NOT RELEIVING with rest and a draining position (with worsening impairment of lymph drainage capacity and of the immunohistochemical alterations of lymph nodes, lymph vessels, and the extracellular matrix).
Type 2 proximal: Where edema is observed at the level of the root of the limb (pitting is rarely positive),
Type 3 distal: At the level of the toes, foot and/or ankle and/o distal part of the calf, pitting is absent and tissues with lymphostatic skin changes are fibrous,
Type 4: lymphedema ("column shaped") at the level of the foot, ankle, calf, knee, and distal parts of the thigh,
Type 5: lymphedema, with sclero-indurative pachydermatis, papillomatous lymphostatic verrucosis: Properly called elephantiasis.
These "typological" definitions will also be used to define the different segments of the limb as defined later (see **Figure 1**) for abnormalities observed on LySc.

Table 2.
The BeSL "clinical" classification-staging-typology of the lower limb lymph-edemas (LLLE).

When faced with patient reporting symptoms that may suggest lower limb lymphedema, the members of the BeSL prefer to report based on clinical findings and use the following typological approach and classification (**Tables 2** and **3**).

3. The lymphoscintigraphies (LySc)

3.1 Introduction to lymphoscintigraphic images

In the field of lymphatic system imaging techniques, lymphoscintigraphies hold a special place. The basic principle is simple: If a radio-labeled molecule (called here "the tracer") injected into a tissue is of sufficient size to enter the lymphatic system, it can be visualized using dedicated gamma cameras to produce static and/or dynamic images, pictures limited to a part of the human body, and/or images of the whole body. The gamma-cameras can also provide three-dimensional images of the distribution of the labeled molecule in the tissues (known as Single Photon Emission Computed Tomography or SPECT) and can be coupled with a X-ray CT scan to position lymphatic structures relative to adjacent organs (known as SPECT-CT) [25–27].

If these nuclear medicine imaging techniques thus result in "qualitative" information about the anatomy of the lymphatic system studied, it must be kept in mind that these

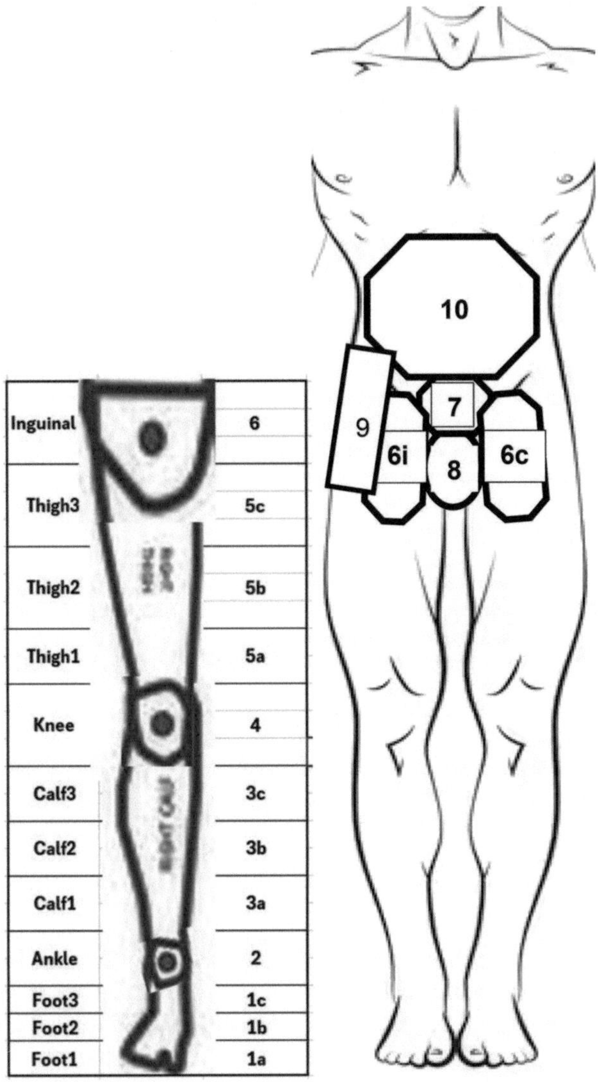

Figure 1.
Segmentation of lower limb and abdomino-pelvic region for defining the localization of lymphatic vascular anomalies.

images are based on the measurement of point signals related to the gamma radiation of radio-elements attached to tracer molecules. Therefore, lymphoscintigraphy exams inherently contain information that is easily quantifiable and quantitative.

In Belgium, the methodology is based on the results of the three-phase lymphoscintigraphic examination developed by the first author of this chapter [7]. This methodology has been adopted since 2009 by Belgian healthcare system to define an edema as lymphatic in origin, as a "lymphedema" [19], and is recommended and supported by BelNuc, the Belgian Society of Nuclear Medicine [28].

However, the experience that the authors of this chapter have with these examinations unfortunately reveals, in a certain number of cases, an incorrect understanding of these images and their contributions. This situation explains why the members of the BeSL find it necessary to review and clarify in this chapter both the methodology of the examination, its images, and their interpretations.

M0: no edema
M0f: no edema but tissue are only "fatty"
M1: no clinical edema, edema diagnosed on para-clinical exam
M2a: pitting is present but less than 1 mm depth
M2b: pitting is present 1–2 mm depth
M2c: pitting is present more than 3 mm depth
Additional annotations:
M1v: tissue are edematous and pitting is present around cutaneous lesions associated to venous disorders
M le-: pitting does not subside with elevation
M i+: with inflammation
M d+: with pain
M ly+: with serous/lymphatic effusion
M or+: with "orange skin" aspect
M3: tissues are hard and fibrous
M4: elephantiasic skin with thickenings, hyperpigmentation, tissue is hard, with increased kinfolds

Table 3.
The BeSL "M-clinical" classification-staging-typology of the lower limb lymph-edemas (LLLE).

3.2 The "three phases" methodological protocol adopted by the Belgian Society of Nuclear Medicine

The methodological protocol can be summarized as follows. 0.2 ml of 99mTc-labeled (74–111 MBq per injection) Human Serum Albumin nanosized colloids (740–1110 MBq of 99 m-TcO4 in 2.0 ml are added in one vial of the product, Nanocoll ® or NanoScint ®) are injected subcutaneously (using tuberculin syringe) in the upper third of the first interdigital space of each foot the patient lying on the table of examination and having been informed that she had not to move the toes and feet during the following 30 minutes.

One static picture of the injected sites is obtained directly after the injections and thereafter the camera head moved on the inguinal areas on which one dynamic imaging is performed (during 30 minutes) in order to see—in resting conditions—the ability of the initial lymphatic system to extract the tracer and to transport it toward the inguinal LN, to estimate the time to inguinal nodes appearance (normally seen after 30 minutes) and to evaluate the possible LV). One first whole body scan-imaging (WBS: anterior and posterior views) is thereafter obtained (this is the "phase 1").

For the "phase 2," one dynamic imaging (lasting 15 minutes) is performed on the inguino-iliac areas but with patient performing tip-toeing during the 15 minutes of the acquisition (the patient still lying on the table of examination) and with the same goals as for "phase 1" (with the tip-toeing, the tracer must move in the LV) but also to have one higher activity in the lymphatic vessels of the limbs. One 2nd WBS is thereafter systematically obtained as well as one 3rd after 1 hour of normal wandering-activities ("phase 3") (see **Figure 2** for a normal LySc-exam). The injected sites are also imaged

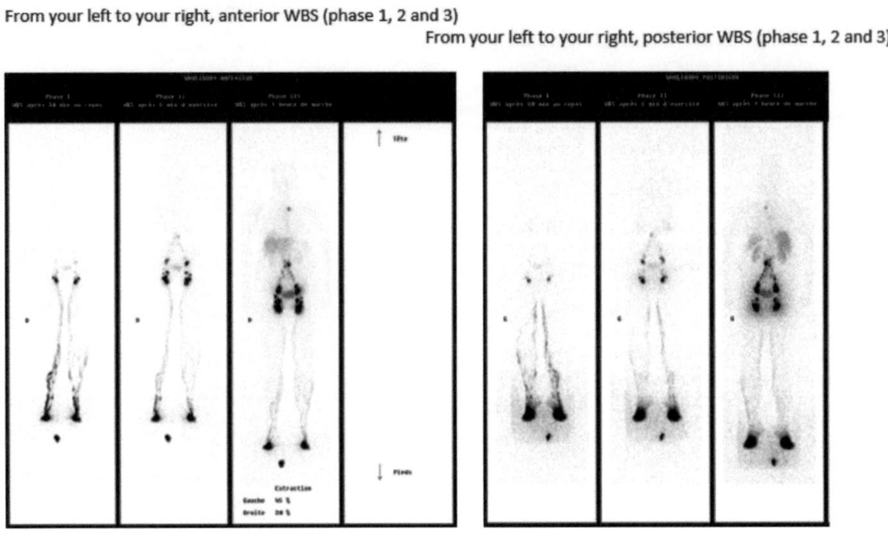

Figure 2.
Normal "3 phase" Lymphoscintigraphy with multiple lymphatic vessels at the level of the feet and calves (with internal and external lymphatic vessels at the level of the left limb), with extraction at the lowest limit on the left (30%) and with one left side retro-clavicula lymph node terminating normally the Ductus Thoracicus (leading thereafter to the normal and delayed visualization of colloidal accumulation in the liver and spleen).

at the end of exam in order to calculate the percent of radio-colloids extracted from the injected sites by the lymphatic system (normal values of extraction are equal or higher than 30%).

The three whole body images (WBS) of each patient are analyzed with at least two contrasts optimized to bring out the signals.

In such LySc investigations, the absence of visualization of some LNs could be normally expected in secondary LLLE (after surgical removal and/or due to fibrosis after surgery and/or radiotherapy) and in primary LLLE (in the case of lymphadeno-aplasia).

When possible, it is recommended to investigate the lymphatic drainage of the root of these limbs. Performing an intradermal injection of radiocolloids in such cases makes it possible to demonstrate the persistence of lymph nodes and the presence of collateral drainage pathways (superficial and/or deep), all of which are useful information for surgeons and/or physiotherapists [29].

Where SPECT-CT devices are available, lympho-SPECT-CT acquisitions should be systematically planned when possible.

3.3 About "morphological" definitions to be used when analyzing the LySc investigations of the lower limbs

3.3.1 The lymph vessels

3.3.1.1 Initial lymphatic vessels (iLV)

Initial lymphatic vessels are exceptionally visible in standard lymphoscintigraphic imaging. They can be visualized when image magnification systems such as "pinholes" are used [30].

3.3.1.2 The superficial cutaneous collateralization network (SCN)

The superficial dermal collateralization network is represented by a honeycomb mesh of small subcutaneous lymphatic vessels, which are primarily characterized by being valveless. This network is connected to adjacent superficial and deep collecting lymphatics. Lymph can progress in all directions within it.

3.3.1.3 Distal "dermal" diffusion through the SCN (dDiffLF)

"Distal dermal diffusion" and progression image defines those images where the tracer from the injection point appears to progress and diffuse through the subcutaneous tissues without any lymphatic vessels being clearly identifiable. In these cases, there is partial progression through the superficial dermal collateralization network. At the periphery of these territories, the tracer may appear in collecting vessels.

3.3.1.4 Collecting lymphatic vessels (LV)

Collecting lymphatic vessels transport lymph and injected radiocolloids that exit the injection point. They produce a linear or more or less convoluted image on static, dynamic, or whole-body images. A "primary" lymphatic vessel efferent to an injection point or several may emerges solely, but they may also divide into multiple "secondary" vessels, which can themselves divide into "tertiary" vessels...

Notes

r.3.3.1.4.1 Their level of definition, our ability to identify them as such, depends on the activity, the radioactive signal, that transits through them.

r.3.3.1.4.2 They are generally clear and identifiable immediately after a phase of tip-toeing exercise.

r.3.3.1.4.3 After a period of walking, they may be less apparent, and their visualization then requires technical adjustments in contrast to the acquired images.

r.3.3.1.4.4 Several lymphatic vessels may "emerge" from injection points and follow parallel or divergent paths.

3.3.1.5 The "collateral lymphatic vessels" (collLV) versus the "lymphatic vessels reflux" (rLV)

A collateral lymphatic is a secondary lymphatic vessel that appears along the path of a primary-main collecting lymphatic vessel and extends superficially in another direction, toward an adjacent cutaneous territory and/or into the depth of the traversed tissues. We propose using "collateral lymphatic vessel" (collLV) when the tracer has not flowed in the superficial network. We distinguish from these collateral vessels (where the tracer progression is normal and related to a simple variant in their anatomical development) from lymphatic vascular refluxes (rLV) that appear secondary to an intra-vascular or intra-nodal lesion leading to this abnormal back-flow progression of the lymph.

3.3.2 The localization-anatomical definition of the normal superficial lymphatic vessels (LV) of the lower limb (LL)

Any tracer injected for lymphatic imaging in the first interdigital space of the foot is normally collected in the medial LV of the dorsum of the foot and, from the region of the malleoli, is transported in the (medial and lateral) LV of the ventromedial

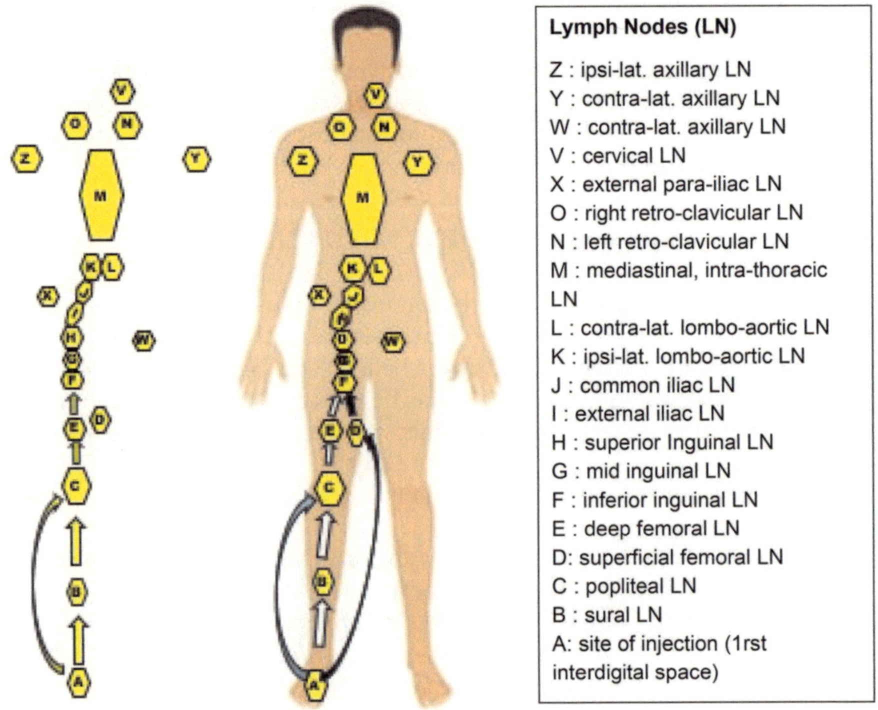

Figure 3.
The LN on the whole body scan after one-side injection in the foot. Arrows (in blue) show the lymph vessels pathways.

(anterior pre-fascial) bundle (also called internal saphenous lymphatics) within 5 to 10 LVs and 4 to 6 main collectors to reach the inguinal lymph nodes at the root of the limb (see **Figure 3**).

Their pathways, however, appear variable and their images are often misinterpreted. These variants are as follows:

a. The LV(s) ascend along the inner part of the calf and thigh.

b. The LV(s) ascend pre-tibial along the leg but return internally below the knee before ascending along the inner part of the thigh.

c. Several LVs ascend from the injection point on the anterior surface of the limb, both internally and externally, at the level of the calf and thigh. This third (and least common) has so far been very rarely associated with clinical edema in the lower limbs but is frequently interpreted as abnormal by some nuclear medicine specialists.

3.3.3 The dermal back-flows (DBF)

3.3.3.1 The dermal backflows in the medical literature

For the 3 imaging techniques of the lymphatic system (Lympho-Scintigraphy, Near-Infra-Red-Fluorescence-Lymphangiography, Magnetic-Resonance

Lymphangiography), the diagnosis of lymphedema is based on the demonstration of dermal reflux of the "tracer" in superficial collateralization lymphatic network, also called "dermal back flow" (DBF). The term appeared in the medical literature devoted to lymphatic vessel imaging of lymphedematous situations as early as 1955 with radiological lymphography [20, 21].

The authors distinguished from the outset:

- proximal reflux (pDBF) following lymph node excision and associated treatments (2ary) and/or congenital lymph-adeno-aplasia (1ary) and/or progressive fibrosis of the inguinal and/or intra-abdominal lymph node structures
- distal reflux (dDBF) following lymphangio-hypo-plasia or lymphangio-hypo-aplasia of the distal lymphatic vessels (initial and/or pre-collectors and/or collectors) in patients who here develop edema that begins in the foot and progresses to the root of the limb.

Between these two extreme developments, segmental dermal back-flows (sDBF) were there after proposed by Browse et al. [22]. These sDBF are considered as "acquired" (rather than congenital) and linked to lymphangio-obliterative phenomena by the development of intraluminal or intramural thrombosis of lymphatic vascular segments. They can be seen in combination with the previous two.

3.3.3.2 The DBF description in the BeSL qualitative analysis

These abnormal lymphatic situations detected on LySc examinations are classified as follows:

- "proximal dermal back flows" (pDBF), that is, images where lymphatic vascular reflux (rLV) at the level of the root of the limb extends to the level of the superficial dermal network and progresses-descends distally until sometimes occurring, reflecting edema affecting the entire lower limb
- "distal dermal back flows" (dDBF), that is, images where rLV begins in the foot, extends to the level of the superficial dermal network to progress upward and until sometimes reflecting edema affecting the entire lower limb
- "Segmental dermal backflow-s" (sDBF), that is, images (where rLV appears between these two extremities of the limb, extends generally to the level of the superficial dermal network and can progress proximally or distally until sometimes showing an edema affecting all or part of the lower limb). The origin of sDBf is defined with reference to "segments" as shown in **Figure 1**.

3.3.4 The lymph nodes (LN)

Lymph nodes are interspersed along the pathways of lymphatic vessels (see **Figure 3**). The injected colloids that pass through these lymph nodes are captured by the reticuloendothelial cells that make up the structure of these lymph nodes. In the context of dynamic imaging of these lymph nodes, it is important to realize that the uptake will occur following a gradient that decreases from the distal part of the limb toward its root and that the uptake of colloids by each lymph node follows a curve with a plateau corresponding to saturation of this uptake by the LN.

One lymph node is thus defined as an active focus interspersed along a lymphatic vascular pathway with the following characteristics:

a. The signal increases over time and does not decrease;

b. The focus must correspond to an anatomical structure dense on CT slices when a SPECT-CT is performed.

Remarks:

r.3.7.1 While superficial lymph nodes (LN) are generally easily identifiable, deep LNs (interspersed in the limbs, intra-abdominal or intra-thoracic) may sometimes be clearer on posterior views than anterior ones, and they will be less clear if their signal is further attenuated by overlying tissue structures (as in subjects with significant overweight).

r.3.7.2 An intense active focus does not mean a large-sized-LN ...

r.3.7.3 A large "sized" LN (palpable or with increased dimensions on SPECT-CT slices) can be inflammatory (or pathological in the case of concomitant lymphomatous disease) and hypo-active.

r.3.7.4 In the context of cancer, all or part of the invaded node-s may not take up the tracer and are not seen, while the healthy part remains visible ...

3.3.4.1 The superficial LV drainage of the lower limbs and their associated LN

Exceptionally, superficial lymph nodes can be observed interspersed at the level of the inner part of the calf.

More frequently observed are the superficial popliteal LN near the opening of the small saphenous vein. The afferent LV of these superficial popliteal LN originate in the lateral surface of the foot and the middle of the calf. These LV form the dorsolateral bundle and are on the surface of the fascia in the distal third of the calf, in the duplication of the fascia in the middle third and beneath the fascia in the proximal third with some superficial collaterals connected to the ventromedial bundle. These superficial popliteal LN are also connected to the deep ones so that all popliteal LN can be detected by filling the superficial nodes and the dorsolateral bundle [18].

LN can also be seen intercalated along the lymphatic vascular pathway in the inner and upper third part of the thigh. Their visualization is not abnormal.

3.3.4.2 The deep-popliteal LN of/draining the lower limbs

The deep-popliteal LN are described medial to the popliteal artery on both side of it (between and/or above the femoral condyles, intercondylar, and/or supracondylar). They receive the lymph from the toes, the muscles of the foot, and lower leg thorough LV accompanying their arteries with intercalated LN at the level of the calf on these deep LV.

Important remarks:

- when the colloids are injected in the first interdigital space of non-edematous feet, the visualization of popliteal LN is abnormal, corresponding to a re-routing of the lymph load and represents one compensatory phenomenon. In our experience, these patients report symptoms of "heavy" limb-s, of edema at the level of ankle and pitting sign may be present in the pre-tibial area.

- On the other hand, in patients without edema, their visualization may be normal when the colloids are injected in the third and/or fourth interdigital space-s and/or in the internal part of the foot.

3.3.5 The inguinal LN

The inguinal lymph nodes can be divided into three groups: inferior, middle, and superior (located at the inguinal canal and connecting with the iliac LN chain). The inferior and middle inguinal lymph nodes receive lymph from both the superficial and deep lymphatic vessels of the leg and thigh.

In an "ideal" schematic presentation, the inguinal lymph nodes would appear on lymphoscintigraphy images as a group of adjacent and "homogeneous" foci, and in its simplest form, like "beads" strung together. In practice, the image is often discontinuous, with well-visualized active lower nodes, less prominent or sometimes absent "middle" nodes, and superior nodes with variable activity.

3.3.6 The intra-abdominal LN

These intra-abdominal lymph nodes (external iliac, common iliac, and lumbo-aortic) should be analyzed on both anterior and posterior images. In individuals with significant overweight, they may appear less clear on the anterior view and more identifiable on the posterior view.

Notes

3.3.6.1 The internal iliac LN (also called "hypogastric") are normally never seen after injections of radio-colloids in the feet.

3.3.6.2 When only one limb is injected, it is normal to see ipsilateral and contralateral lumbo-aortic LN because they are interconnected.

3.3.7 The ductus thoracicus and the intra-thoracic LN

We have extensively analyzed the presence of supradiaphragmatic lymph nodes in the context of lymphoscintigraphy of the lower limbs and reported the results in one of our articles [31].

While the visualization of nodes in the left retro-clavicular space is well-known and normal, it must also be considered that nodes can be interspersed along the path of the normal thoracic duct, as well as on its "collaterals" related to variants associated with a "malformation" during its embryonic development.

3.3.8 The collateralization of LV

The collateralization of LV pathways at the level of the root of the limb from the thigh and/or from the inguinal area can be seen pre-pubic toward the contra-lateral, toward the genital area, the magna labia for the woman, the scrotum and penis for the man, from down (the pelvis) to up (the supra-diaphragmatic LN as the axillary ones, the para-sternal ones), toward the external part of the buttock, and toward the posterior and/or lateral part of the abdominal wall.

3.3.9 LN intercalated

LN intercalated on the collateralization pathways from the root of the limb can also sometimes be seen: (the most frequent) above the iliac crest-bone, beyond the femoral bone, intra-muscular inter-gluteal, above and around the iliac crest-bone, between the epigastric anterior muscles, pre-sacral, para-renal, intercostal and para-vertebral, para-retro-sternal ("internal mammary," sometimes with the pre-pericardic LN), latero-thoracic ("external mammary"), and in the axillary area.

3.4 About our analysis of "morpho-functional" parameters

3.4.1 The time to node in resting conditions (phase 1) in the BeSL index

The time to node, which analyzes the arrival of the tracer at the inguinal nodes, depends on several factors: the capacity of the initial lymphatics to absorb the colloids, the lymphatic load at the injected tissues, and the ability of the lymphatic vessels to transport the tracer to these nodes at the root of the limb. Within the framework of our lymphoscintigraphic protocol, the arrival of the tracer is considered normal if observed within 30 minutes following the injection. The time to node should be interpreted in relation to the subject's biological context: It will be "faster" in cases of heart failure, renal failure, or hypo-proteinemia.

It may be abnormal if:

- Tissue and/or lymphatic changes at the injection site are such that the tracer stagnates there,
- Lymphatic lesions are observed.

A very rapid arrival (within 5–10 minutes following the injection) can sometimes be observed. It is important first to ensure that the injection was indeed subcutaneous and not intradermal (with the formation of a tense local papule). Such rapid arrivals in the context of the limb should raise suspicion of one of the following situations at the injection site:

- An anomaly in the venous return of the limb and/or
- A hyperemic inflammatory process at the distal part of the limb and/or
- A deep lymphatic network that is hypo-functional or non-functional, resulting in rerouting of the deep lymphatic load to the superficial network.

3.4.2 The analysis of tracer accumulation in lymph nodes during the tip-toeing exercise (phase 2)

Performing tip-toeing for 5 to 15 minutes (phase 2) leads to the opening of the initial lymphatic junctions, the entry of interstitial fluids and the tracer into the

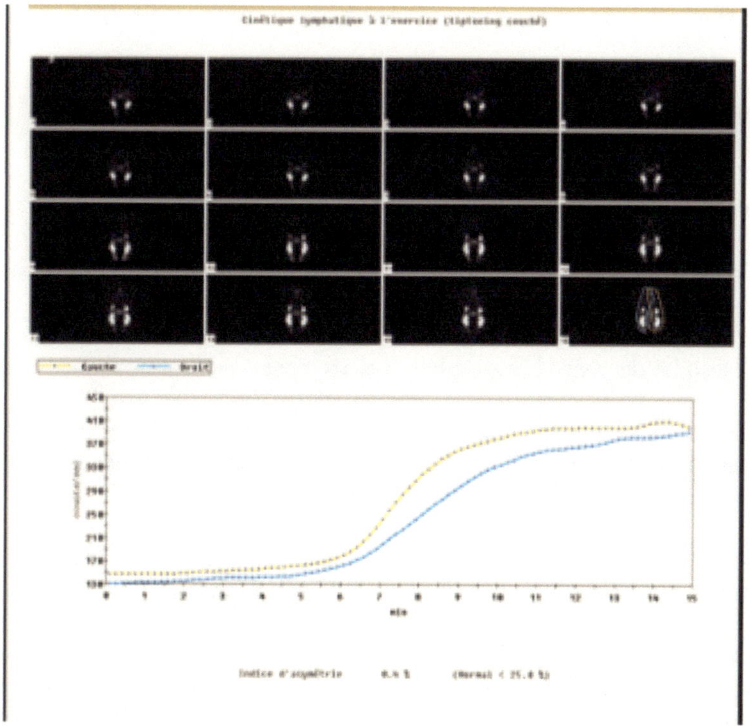

Figure 4.
Dynamic imaging centered on the inguinal areas during 15 minutes with tip-toeing from the 6th to the 10th minutes and the time activity curves generated from areas of interest drawn on and including all the visualized Lymph Nodes.

collecting lymphatics, their loading, the activation of their contractions (also within the framework of underlying tissue movements), and the propulsion of the tracer into the lymph nodes where it penetrates and is partially accumulated with kinetics per node reaching a plateau corresponding to its saturation.

In the case of normal limbs, the kinetics of activities in the LN and their curves (when compared) are "parallel" (see **Figure 4**) with an -normal- asymmetry that should not exceed a 25% difference from the average of their sums in terms of total accumulated activity (in all the LN seen) at the end of the examination.

In some cases, a curve may not show a plateau but rather a decrease after reaching a maximum. This situation is observed when there is an intra-nodal lymphatic-venous shunt. It corresponds to the drainage of the nodal content of the tracer by the nodal veins, and at the same time, a signal may appear in the liver. This situation occurs in the case of a nodal block upstream.

Note: A frequently observed error in these analysis is drawing the region of interest (ROI) on only one (often the first) inguinal lymph node. This ROI should cover all lymph nodes observed at the end of this phase.

3.4.3 The activities in the inguino-Ilio-lumbo-aortic LN (phase 3)

Similarly, the presence of LN, the activity seen in the inguino-ilio-lumbo-aortic lymph nodes (and when present in the intra-thoracic LN) and in the liver, should be understood as follows:

- The observed activity depends on what has been able to exit from the injection site,
- It will be higher when the lymphatic system is normal,
- It will be lower when the conditions at the injection site are such that extraction is further reduced,
- It will also be lower when anomalies in tracer distribution are observed (more or less extensive DBF),
- It will also be decreased if lymph nodes are observed “intercalated” in the limb.

It should be noted that factors such as a subject’s obesity will provide an attenuated image of the ilio-lumbo-aortic lymph nodes and hepatic activity without allowing for “pathological” conclusions to be drawn.

3.4.4 Visualization of the liver (and sometimes the spleen and more rarely the bone marrow): The whole-body lymph system colloidal index?

Visualization of activity in the liver and spleen and sometimes the bone marrow is normal. It corresponds to the uptake of colloids by the reticuloendothelial cells of these organs, to the part of the colloids that have traveled from the foot through the entire lymphatic vascular axis to the opening in the left subclavian vein AND that have not been captured in the lymph nodes themselves.

r.3.4.4.1 It is not normal to visualize hepato-spleno-medullary activity on phase 1 WBS. This image most often results from an intravenous (IV) injection of colloids at one or both feet. Residual venous transit above the foot or on the first pictures of the dynamic acquisition centered on the inguinal nodes may also then suggest this IV injection.

r.3.4.4.2 Hepatic activity may sometimes be observed on phase 2 or 3 images when the tracer has reached only the inguinal nodes WITHOUT the overlying nodes being observed. This image should then suggest the presence of an intra-nodal lymphatico-venous shunt [32].

3.5 BeSL transport index (severity score) classification for LLLE based on the interpretation of the 3-phase LySc (BeSL LLLE-SS v3:07/2025)

Based on the images from three-phase lymphoscintigraphy examinations of the lower limbs, it is proposed to calculate an evaluation score of the lymphatic situation. This index is inspired by the one proposed by Kleinhans et al. [5]. It is certainly more complex but more comprehensive, taking into account various parameters not clearly addressed by these authors. The value of this score (resulting from the summation of the different parameters listed below) will be higher as the lymphatic condition is more advanced or deteriorated.

This index has prognostic value regarding the progression of the clinical situation and can be used to monitor the response to treatment.

This index (like the TNM of various cancers) will likely be subject to adaptations as new studies will published, analyzing its prognostic and/or predictive values in various forms of lower limb lymphedema.

3.5.1 The "functional" parameters

3.5.1.1 "Time to" inguinal LN

0 = Inferior inguinal LN are well seen after phase 1 and activities in the LN are symmetric

1 = Inferior inguinal LN are faintly seen after phase 1

+1 = Inferior inguinal LN are seen after phase 1 but activities in the LN are asymmetric ➔ value +1 is given to the limb with the lowest activity

2 = Inferior inguinal LN are seen only after phase 2 and activities in the LN are symmetric

+ 1 is added to the limb with the lowest activity if activities in the LN are asymmetric ➔ value +1 is given to the limb with the lowest activity

= Inguinal and at least iliac LN are seen after phase 3

+ 1 is added to the limb with the lowest activity when activities in the LN are asymmetric ➔ value +1 is given to the limb with the lowest activity

10 = Inguinal and iliac LN are not seen after phase ➔ value +10 is given to the limb without LN

3.5.1.2 "Superficial LV (sLV) at the level of the limb"

0 = sLV are well seen bilaterally after phases 1, 2, and 3 and activities in the LV are symmetric µ

1 = sLV are faintly seen after phase 1

+1 = if activities in the LV are asymmetric after phase 1 ➔ value +1 is given to the limb with the lowest activity

2 = sLV are seen only after phase 2

+1 = if activities in the LV are asymmetric after phase 2 ➔ value +1 is given to the limb with the lowest activity

3 = sLV are seen only on WBS after phase 3

+1 = if activities in the LV are asymmetric after phase 3 ➔ value +1 is given to the limb with the lowest activity

+5 if sLV are faintly seen after phase ➔ value +5 is given to the limb with the lowest activity

+10 if sLV are not seen after phase 3 ➔ value +10 is given to the limb without sLV visualization

3.5.1.3 Popliteal LN and deep LV-L drainage

+6 if pop LN are seen after phase 1

+4 if pop LN are seen after phase 2

+2 if pop LN are only seen and clear after phase 3

+1 if pop LN are only seen but faint on spect-ct after phase 3

3.5.1.4 Activities in the inguino-Ilio-lumbo-aortic LN and in liver

0 if LN are seen after phase 1 and activities are symmetric

+1 = if activities in the LN are asymmetric ➔ value +1 is given to the limb with the lowest activity

+2 if LN are not seen after phase 1
0 if activities are increasing symmetrically after phase 2
+1 = activity does not increase at the level of one limb
+1 = if the increase of the activities in the LN are asymmetric ➔ value +1 is given to the limb with the lowest activity
+ 3 if LN are not seen after phase 2 ➔ value +1 is given to the limb without LN

Activities are increasing symmetrically after phase 3
+1 = activity does not increase at the level of one limb (added to the limb without increase)
+1 = if the increase of the activities in the LN are asymmetric ➔ value +1 is given to the limb with the lowest activity
+ 6 if LN are not seen after phase 3 ➔ value is given to the limb without LN

+ 20 if intra-abdominal LN are not seen after phase 2 and/or 3 on one side
+ 40 if intra-abdominal LN are not seen after phase 2 and/or 3 on both side

3.5.1.5 Extraction (E.)

0 if extraction at the end of the exam is normal (= or > 30%)
+3 if extractions are higher than 30% but asymmetric (see 3.4.2) ➔ value +1 is given to the limb with the lowest E
+1 if extraction is under 30% but higher than 24%
+2 if extraction is under 25% but higher than 19
+4 if extraction is under 20% but higher than 14%
+7 if extraction is under 15% but higher than 9%
+11 if extraction is under 10%

3.5.1.6 The dermal back flow-s in our VLM index

We consider the presence and location of these DBFs as one of the important factors in our classification, and we therefore have five situations leading to five corresponding indexes:

- An index for cases without DBF
- An index for pure dDBF
- An index for pure pDBF
- An index for isolated sDBF
- An index for mixed situations

3.5.2 BeSL transport index (severity score) classification for LLLE with sDBF on LySc

+ 10 per sDBF level identified on LySc

+ 5 if segmental rLV at the origin-responsible of the sDBF is identified after phase 1
+ 3 if segmental rLV at the origin-responsible of the sDBF is identified after phase 2
+ 1 if segmental rLV at the origin-responsible of the sDBF is identified after phase 3
+ 4 per additional segment above and/or under the original segment

3.5.3 BeSL transport index (severity score) classification for LLLE with dDBF on LySc

per dDBF level identified on LySc
+ 20 if dDBF is identified after phase 1
+ 10 if dDBF is identified after phase 2
+ 5 if dDBF is identified only after phase 3

+ per segment progression only at the level of the foot
+2 if only distal third of the foot
+4 if mid part of the foot
+6 if the whole foot

+ 8 if progression at the ankle
…

+20 if progression up to the groin

3.5.4 BeSL transport index (severity score) classification for LLE with pDBF on LySc

+ 20 if pDBF is identified after phase 1
+ 10 if pDBF is identified after phase 2
+ 5 if pDBF is identified after phase 3

+ 2 per segment distal progression toward the foot
+ 4 per segment progression at the homo- and/or hetero-lateral (buttock) and/or "upward" (pelvis, abdomen, …) part-s of the body

3.5.5 LN and/or LN "aplasia-hypoplasia" in the BeSL transport index (severity score) classification

3.5.3.1 After interdigital injection *for the patients with suspected primary LLE*, only deep lymphatic vessels (dLV) are seen at the level of the calf with intercalated lymph nodes, sometimes without inferior inguinal LN: superficial lymph-angio-aplasia or sLVA ➔ +20

3.5.3.2 After interdigital injection for the patients with suspected primary LLE, inguinal and/or iliac LN are not seen: "Lympho-Nodal-Aplasia" (or LNA) ➔ +5 per LN "groups" as defined in **figure 3**

3.5.5.3 After injection [18] in the retro malleolar anterior space of the triceps surae tendon (Kager's triangle), no deep lymph vessels are seen running deep in the calf: sometimes with increased lymph flow at the level of the superficial LV of the edematous limb when compared to the normal limb (10): deep lympho-nodal " aplasia " or dLNA ➔ +5

3.5.5.4 After interdigital injection for all patients, both deep and superficial LVs are observed with popliteal and/or sural intercalated LN: "superficial and/or deep lymph-angio hypoplasia" or sLVH-dLVH ➔ +5

3.5.5.5 After interdigital injection, inguinal and/or iliac LN are seen hypoactive at the level of the limb-s (see **Figure 3**): "Lympho-Nodal-Hypoplasia" (or LNH) ➔ +1 (per limb)

3.5.5.6 After interdigital injection for all patients, the tracer does not reach the inferior inguinal LN after phase 1 (See **Figure 2**) and/or after phase 2 and/or extraction is decreased under the value of 30% and/or extractions, nodal accumulations of the tracer after phase 1 and/or 2 (see **Figure 2**) show significant asymmetry: "Lymph-System-Hypoplasia" or LSH ➔ +5

3.5.5.7 After interdigital injection for all patients, inguinal and iliac LN are well seen but pLVR are seen: "proximal Lympho-Nodal-Hypoplasia" (or pLNH) ➔ +10 per limb with pLVR.

3.5.6 Regarding the "specificity" of the different parameters of this index?

In our first series of studies on normal limbs [7], we observed that among 20 young (age under 30 years old) and healthy subjects with limbs without edema and presumed normal, the "time to node" after phase 1 was abnormal for one limb in just one case, and the extraction at the end of the examination was equal to or greater than 30% for all subjects. In a recent series of 60 young volunteers without edema in their lower limbs (unpublished data), the investigation of their lymphatic systems suggested the presence of deep lymphatic drainage from the injection point in two cases. This observation suggests that "abnormal" variants might be present, latent, and "innate" in a small percentage of cases. Additionally in a recent retrospective review of 41 patients (mean age = 51.1 years, range 24–75 years) who were identified in our database who had been operated for one melanoma at the level of one lower limb and undergone routine, clinically indicated lymphoscintigraphy when they developed lower limb edema at the level of their operated limb but no symptom and/or sign at the level of their non-operated one (unpublished data), popliteal LN were seen in four cases (in 10% of the limbs), the tracer did not reach the first inguinal lymph nodes in 11 out of 41 cases (or 27%: by the end of phase 1, in 6 out of 15 or 40% for left limbs, and in 5 out of 26 or 19% for right limbs) and the extraction was abnormal in 8 subjects out of 41 (or 25% but for 5 of 15 left limbs or 33% and 3 of 26 right or 11.5%). These observations in this series may appear somewhat "disturbing" if it is not hypothesized that these anomalies are observed in subjects who developed edema in the operated lower limb. These anomalies in their non-operated limb might actually indicate a pre-existing latent insufficiency in their lymphatic system revealed by the operation.

3.6 Summary of the approach for using the BeSL VLM (-TNM like) "classifications" of the lower limb lymph-edemas

Our classification of lower limb lymphedema (LLLE) corresponds to a logical and rational "sequential" approach that is based first on clinical data and then on the results of imaging examinations of the lymphatic system.

(1) Step 1: Consider that there are several different types of lymphedema based on the clinic (see **Table 1**).

See **Table 4**.

Step 1	Syndromic	1ary	2ary	Lipedema	NOC
		Congenital	Ca. Rel. L		
		Praecox	Phlebo. L		
		Tarda	Neuro. L		

Step 1	Syndromic	1ary	2ary	Lipedema	NOC
		" sporadic "	Inf. L		
		" familial "	Bone Arth. L		
			Syst. Dis L		

Table 4.
The BeSL "clinical" classification of the lower limb lymph-edemas (LLLE).

(2) Step 2: Then consider that the location and clinical extent of the edema represent different situations (see § 2.2.1 "From T-nm to V-lm" and **Figure 1**).

See **Table 5**.

Step 2	Vd	Vp	Vs1	VsX	Vw

Table 5.
Definitions of the location and extent of the edema (see § 2.1.1).

(3) Step 3a: Take into account the classification of these edemas proposed by the ISL, particularly in aspects corresponding to tissue changes.

See **Table 6**.

Step 3a	ISL St. 0	ISL St. 1	ISL St. 2 early	ISL St. 2 late	ISL St. 3

Table 6.
ISL classification of the LLE (1).

Step 3b: Apply the BeSL Classification ("Typology") for the tissues of the edematous limb (see **Tables 2** and **3**).

See **Table 7**.

Step 3b Segments?	BeSL «type » 0	BeSL « type » 1 Distal Segmental	BeSL « type » 2 Distal Segmental Proximal	BeSL « type » 3 Distal	BeSL « type » 4	BeSL « Type » 5

Table 7.
*BeSL Classification for the tissues of the edematous limbs (see **Tables** 2 and 3).*

(4) Step 4: *When no DBF is observed*, we arrive at a classification based on the images of lymphatic vessels (LV) and lymph nodes (LN) within the framework of their sequential appearance as proposed in the 3-phase approach.

See **Table 8**.

Step 4: LV and/or LN A or Hypo "Plasia" →	sLVA*	sLVH – dLVH	LNA*	LNH	LSH	Deep LL LNA*	pLNH

use specifically the term "aplasia" to describe the lymphatic structures when primary LLLE are suspected.

Table 8.
Lymph Vessel and/or Lymph Node Aplasia or Hypoplasia Classification (see § 2.1.2).

(5) Step 5: Then base your approach on the absence or presence of dermal backflow (DBF) on lympho-scintigraphic images (see **Figure 1** to determine-define the segment-s and their extension-s).

See **Table 9**.

Step 4	**No DBF**	**dDBF**	**pDBF**	**sDBF**	**mDBF**

Table 9.
About Dermal Back-Flows (see § 3.3.3.2).

(6) Step 6: our Transport Index / Severity Score can then be used in our analytical grid for LLLE (see **Table 10**): Faced with the lymphoscintigraphic images of a patient, record your observations in **Table 10**, sum the numbers, and you will obtain the Severity Score according to the BeSL.

	Group?							
	ISL?		BeSL?		ISL?		BeSL?	
	V?				V?			
	Right LL			LV-LN A-/Hypo "plasia"	Left LL			LV-LN A-/Hypo "plasia"
	Ph1	Ph2	Ph3		Ph1	Ph2	Ph3	
Time to Ing LN								
sLV								
Deep L (pop LN)								
Extraction								
pDBF								
sDBF								
dDBF								
Sum								
Conclusion								

Table 10.
Analytical grid proposed to be used for LLLE (BeSL LLLE LySc v3-27,072,025).

4. Conclusions

The medical management of patients presenting with edema of one or both lower limbs has given rise to numerous articles with varied data, the reading of which often leaves even the most persistent readers with an impression of "chaos." This literature is also often lacking in details, as well as in clear (images and) definitions. In the chapter developed here for this book, members of the Belgian Society of Lymphology revisit, clarify, and detail the methodology adopted by the Belgian Society of Nuclear Medicine for imaging lower limb edema (and by Belgian healthcare authorities for defining these edemas as lymphedemas and for the reimbursement of their treatments). The definitions of the images thus obtained for the various structures composing the lymphatic system are specified and detailed, along with useful remarks for their proper use. Different terms frequently used in the workup of these edemas (such as aplasia, hypoplasia, dermal reflux …) are precised. This methodological approach also provides functional information, which is likewise detailed and clarified with useful comments for appropriate application. Just as there is not one cancer but many cancers, the members of the Belgian Society of Lymphology also consider that there is not one lymphedema but many lymphedemas, each of which should be considered as a unique and singular entity. They therefore propose the so-called "VLM" classification of this form of lymphedemas, analogous to the TNM classification for cancers. Ultimately, this results in what we believe to be a more rational approach to these edematous situations, both for use by front-line clinicians in their diagnostic workup and by therapists who will subsequently manage them [33–39].

Author details

Pierre Bourgeois[1,2,3]*, Mirela Mariana Roman[4], Romain Barbieux[5], Joseph Harfouche[6] and Olivier Leduc[5]

1 Service of Dermatology, Hospital Erasme, Université Libre de Bruxelles, Brussels, Belgium

2 Service of Vascular Surgery, HIS-IZZ Hospitals, Université Libre de Bruxelles, Brussels, Belgium

3 Services of Nuclear Medicine, Institute Jules Bordet and HIS-IZZ Hospitals, Université Libre de Bruxelles, Brussels, Belgium

4 Department of Mammo-Pelvic Surgery, CHU St. Pierre, Université Libre de Bruxelles, Brussels, Belgium

5 Department of Occupational and Environmental Physiology, Lympho-phlebology Unit, Haute Ecole, Université Libre de Bruxelles, Brussels, Belgium

6 Department of Physical Therapy, Delta Hospitals, Brussels, Belgium

*Address all correspondence to: pierre.bourgeois2201@gmail.com; pierre.bourgeois@hubruxelles.be

References

[1] Consensus ISL. The diagnosis and treatment of peripheral lymphedema: 2023 consensus document of the International Society of Lymphology. Lymphology. 2024;**56**(4):133-151

[2] Szuba A, Shin WS, Strauss HW, Rockson S. The third circulation: Radionuclide lymphoscintigraphy in the evaluation of lymphedema. Journal of Nuclear Medicine. 2003;**44**:43-57

[3] Weissleder H, Weissleder R. Lymphedema: Evaluation of qualitative and quantitative lymphoscintigraphy in 238 patients. Radiology. 1988;**167**(3): 729-735

[4] Ter SE, Alavi A, Kim CK, Merli G. Lymphoscintigraphy: A reliable test for the diagnosis of lymphedema. Clinical Nuclear Medicine. 1993;**18**:646-654

[5] Kleinhans E et al. Evaluation of transport kinetics in lymphoscintigraphy: Follow-up study in patients with transplanted lymphatic vessels. European Journal of Nuclear Medicine. 1985;**10**(7–8):349-352

[6] Cambria RA, Gloviczki P, Naessens JM, Wahner HW. Noninvasive evaluation of the lymphatic system with lymphoscintigraphy: A prospective, semiquantitative analysis in 386 extremities. Journal of Vascular Surgery. 1993;**18**(5):773-782

[7] Bourgeois P, Munck D, Becker C, Leduc O, Leduc A. A three-phase lymphoscintigraphic investigation protocol for the evaluation of lower limb edemas. The European Journal of Lymphology and Related Problems. 1997;**9**(21):10-21

[8] Williams WH, Witte CL, Witte MH, McNeill GC. Radionuclide lymphangioscintigraphy in the evaluation of peripheral lymphedema. Clinical Nuclear Medicine. 2000;**25**:451-464

[9] Moshiri M, Katz DS, Boris M, Yung E. Using lymphoscintigraphy to evaluate suspected lymphedema of the extremities. AJR. American Journal of Roentgenology. 2002;**178**:405-412

[10] Maccauro M et al. Lymphoscintigraphy for the evaluation of limb lymphatic flow disorders: Report of technical procedural standards from an Italian nuclear medicine expert panel. Revista Espanola De Medicina Nuclear E Imagen Molecular. 2019;**38**(5): 335-340

[11] Keramida G et al. Importance of accurate Ilio-inguinal quantification in lower extremity lymphoscintigraphy. Nuclear Medicine Communications. 2017;**38**(3):209-214

[12] Bourgeois P. Critical analysis of the literature on lymphoscintigraphic investigations of limb edemas. The European Journal of Lymphology and Related Problems. 1997;**9**(21):1-9

[13] Bourgeois P. Radionuclide lymphoscintigraphies. In: Greene AK, Slavin SA, Brörson H, editors. Lymphedema: Presentation, Diagnosis and Treatment. Switzerland: Springer; 2018. pp. 253-263

[14] Brierley JD, Gospodarowicz MK, Wittekind C, editors. TNM Classification of Malignant Tumours. 8th ed. Wiley-Blackwell; 2016

[15] Duhon BH et al. Current mechanistic understandings of lymphedema and lipedema: Tales of fluid, fat, and fibrosis. International Journal of Molecular Sciences. 2022;**23**(12):6621

[16] Markarian B et al. Assessment modalities for lower extremity edema, lymphedema, and lipedema: A scoping review. Cureus. 2024;**16**(3):e55906

[17] Greene AK et al. Obesity-induced lymphedema: Clinical and lymphoscintigraphic features. Plastic and Reconstructive Surgery. 2015;**135**(6):1715-1719

[18] Barbieux R et al. Scintigraphic investigations of the deep and superficial lymphatic systems in the evaluation of lower limb oedema. Scientific Reports. 2019;**9**:13691

[19] INAMI. Circulaire kinésithérapeutes. 2009. 1 annexe 2 [Internet]. Available from: https://www.inami.fgov.be/SiteCollectionDocuments/circulaire_kinesitherapeutes_2009_1_annexe2.pdf and from: https://www.inami.fgov.be/fr/professionnels/professionnels-de-la-sante/kinesitherapeutes/pour-quelles-pathologies-lourdes-votre-patient-peut-il-beneficier-d-un-remboursement-plus-eleve-de-sa-kinesitherapie

[20] Kinmonth JB et al. Lymphangiography: A technique for its clinical use in the lower limb. British Medical Journal. 1955;**1**(4919):940-942

[21] Kinmonth JB et al. Primary lymphedema; clinical and lymphangiographic studies of a series of 107 patients. The British Journal of Surgery. 1957;**45**(189):1-9

[22] Browse NL, Stewart G. Lymphedema: Pathophysiology and classification. The Journal of Cardiovascular Surgery. 1985;**26**(2):91-106

[23] Papendieck CM. Lymphatic dysplasia in pediatrics: A new classification. International Angiology. 1999;**18**(1):6-9

[24] Wolfe JH, Kinmonth JB. The prognosis of primary lymphedema of the lower limbs. Archives of Surgery. 1981;**116**(9):1157-1160. DOI: 10.1001/archsurg.1981.01380210037007

[25] Baulieu F et al. Contributions of SPECT/CT imaging to the lymphoscintigraphic investigations of the lower limb lymphedema. Lymphology. 2013;**46**(3):106-119

[26] Weiss M et al. Primary lymphedema of the lower limb: The clinical utility of single photon emission computed tomography/CT. Korean Journal of Radiology. 2015;**16**(1):188-195

[27] Yoon HJ et al. The added value of SPECT/CT lymphoscintigraphy in the initial assessment of secondary extremity lymphedema patients. Scientific Reports. 2023;**13**:19494

[28] BelNuc. Société belge de médecine nucléaire [Internet]. Available from: https://www.belnuc.be/?s=lymphedema

[29] Bourgeois P, Leduc O. Value of one additional injection at the root of the limb in the lymphoscintigraphic evaluation and management of primary and secondary lower-limb lymphedemas. PLoS One. 2021;**16**(7):e0253900

[30] Lijowski M, Caruthers S, Hu G, Zhang H, Scott MJ, Williams T, et al. High-resolution SPECT-CT/MR molecular imaging of angiogenesis in the Vx2 model. Investigative Radiology. 2009;**44**(1):15-22. DOI: 10.1097/RLI.0b013e31818935eb

[31] Bourgeois P, Munck D, Sales F. Anomalies of thoracic lymph duct drainage demonstrated by lymphoscintigraphy. European Journal of Surgical Oncology. 2008;**34**(5):553-555

[32] Edwards JM, Kinmonth JB. Lymphovenous shunts in man. British Medical Journal. 1969;**4**(5683):579-581

[33] Foeldi M, Foeldi E, Kubik S. Textbook of Lymphology: For Physicians and Lymphedema Therapists. Munchen: Elsevier GmbH; 2003

[34] Moreno Gonzalez E, Olivera DJ. Adenolympho-saphenous anastomosis using the Nielubowicz-Olszewski-Sakolowski method. Angiología. 1972;**24**:5-8

[35] Languasco GB, Cacciatore E, Iachino C. Lymphedema and lymphonodovenous anastomosis. Proposal of a technical modification. Angiología. 1989;**41**:11-16

[36] Allen RJ Jr, Cheng MH. Lymphedema surgery: Patient selection and an overview of surgical techniques. Journal of Surgical Oncology. 2016;**113**: 923-931

[37] Cheng MH, Pappalardo M, Lin C, Kuo C, Lin CY, Chung KC. Validity of the novel Taiwan lymphoscintigraphy staging and correlation of Cheng lymphedema grading for unilateral extremity lymphedema. Annals of Surgery. 2018;**268**:513-525

[38] Baumeister RG, Seifert J, Wiebecke B. Homologous and autologous experimental lymph vessel transplantation: Initial experience. International Journal of Microsurgery. 1981;**3**:19-24

[39] Baumeister RG, Mayo W, Notohamiprodjo M, Wallmichrath J, Springer S, Frick A. Microsurgical Lymphatic Vessel Transplantation. Journal of Reconstructive Microsurgery. 2016;**32**:34-41